SOMEONE WAS HERE

Profiles in the AIDS Epidemic

Also by George Whitmore

THE CONFESSIONS OF DANNY SLOCUM
NEBRASKA

SOMEONE WAS HERE

Profiles in the AIDS Epidemic

George Whitmore

NAL BOOKS

NEW AMERICAN LIBRARY

NEW YORK AND SCARBOROUGH, ONTARIO

NAL TRADEMARK REG. U.S. PAT. OFF. AND FOREIGN COUNTRIES
REGISTERED TRADEMARK—MARCA REGISTRADA
HECHO EN CHICAGO, U.S.A.

SIGNET, SIGNET CLASSIC, MENTOR, ONYX, PLUME, MERIDIAN
and NAL BOOKS are published *in the United States* by NAL PENGUIN INC.,
1633 Broadway, New York, New York 10019,
in Canada by The New American Library of Canada Limited,
81 Mack Avenue, Scarborough, Ontario M1L 1M8

Library of Congress Cataloging-in-Publication Data

Whitmore, George, 1945–
    Someone was here.

    1. AIDS (Disease)—Case studies.   2. AIDS (Disease)
—Social aspects.   3. AIDS (Disease)—Psychological
aspects.   4. AIDS (Disease)—Patients—Family
relationships.   I. Title.
RC607.A26W495   1988   362.1'969792'00924   87-31407
ISBN 0-453-00601-9

Designed by Leonard Telesca

First Printing, April, 1988

    2   3   4   5   6   7   8   9

PRINTED IN THE UNITED STATES OF AMERICA

For Michael, who endured

ACKNOWLEDGMENTS

This book wouldn't have been possible without the generous participation of a score of people who consented to be interviewed at length on their experiences relating to AIDS. Their contribution is abundantly evident in the text. But thanks are also due to dozens of others who shared their knowledge and insight in background interviews.

Many friends and acquaintances too numerous to name supported this work in very material ways and all deserve my gratitude. Susan Kaslow, James Ross Smith, and Mark Hayman, who transcribed tapes for me, made this project feasible. Joan Tedeschi provided valuable research assistance. Jed Mattes, my agent, always had a helping hand extended. Special thanks, as well, to the MacDowell Colony, a safe haven, where most of this book was written.

Portions of this book originally appeared in a different form in *The New York Times Magazine.* My thanks to Gerald Walker for editing with tact and sensitivity. At New American Library, Helen Eisenbach insistently pursued this project and Gary Luke was unusually patient and understanding during its completion. Thanks also to Paul Scanlon for the book title.

The author wishes to acknowledge with gratitude permission to quote from Wilfred Owen's "Insensibility" from the Owen Estate, Chatto & Windus, Ltd., and New Directions Publishing Corp.: *The Collected Poems of Wilfred Owen,* edited by C. Day Lewis, © Chatto & Windus, Ltd., 1946.

AUTHOR'S NOTE

Attempting to define the galvanizing phenomenon—political, social, medical—of AIDS in America is somewhat like the parable about the three blind men and the elephant: one holds in his hand a rope, another works his way along a wall, the third wrestles with a boa constrictor. AIDS is a mirror, reflecting every individual's deepest fears. AIDS is a magnet, indiscriminately attracting all manner of prejudices. AIDS is a juggernaut cutting a wide swath across the nation. This book can only provide a partial view of a few aspects of it. I would have liked to have provided a panorama. But AIDS is moving too fast for that, so I've had to settle for something more like snapshots taken from a speeding train. Consider: this book covers three years in the epidemic. In February 1985, when the book begins, there were 8,495 diagnosed cases of AIDS nationwide. In February 1987, when it ends, there were 31,036.

This book consists primarily of interviews with people who told their stories to me in an effort to further understanding about AIDS and the human tragedy it is. Notwithstanding the potent stigma attached to AIDS, without exception the protagonists of this book insisted on using their real names. In order to protect confidentiality, however, names of patients at Lincoln Hospital have been changed and certain identifying characteristics have been altered. In a few other instances where participants requested that only first names or pseudonyms be used, it's indicated in the text.

Although, obviously, I've dramatized events in this book, it is factual. Conversations and incidents I didn't witness were reconstructed. Some were telescoped and/or streamlined to provide a coherent narrative. Many are based on hearsay—that is, the unconfirmed recollection of a single participant.

CONTENTS

Prologue   1
1985: Greenwich Village, New York City   5
1986: Greeley, Colorado   71
1987: Lincoln Hospital, the South Bronx   125
Epilogue   205

PROLOGUE

There's a picture I keep in front of me. I cut it out of a magazine. It's a photograph taken in a monastery on Mt. Athos, a peninsula in northern Greece. The monasteries at Mt. Athos were founded in Byzantine times and, as far as anyone knows, no woman has set foot on the peninsula since then. So if you're male, you can apply for permission to visit the monks on Mt. Athos, who otherwise live utterly isolated amidst amazing treasures just as they have for centuries.

This photo was taken in a charnel house and the first thing you see is skulls, a pile of them. They're stacked up neatly in rows, one on top of the other. Images of the Black Death come instantly to mind.

One skull is out of place—maybe someone was careless arranging the skulls or maybe the pile settled over the years, for one skull lies face up. Instead of eye- and nose-holes, you find yourself looking into the hole where the spine went in—a round "O"—and the two hollows under the cheekbones. It makes this face look exclamatory.

The skulls sit in ranks on a ledge against a rough whitewashed wall. Some of them are almost as white as the wall. Others are parchment-colored. The pile of skulls is so graphic, at first you don't even notice the monk.

This monk—recedes into the background. He's wearing black. The photographer's flash casts the wall behind him into shadow. His black beard all but obscures a gaunt profile. He's holding a big box full of bones.

The box is made of wood and has a hinged lid. There are two skulls and some arm or shin bones in the box. One of the skulls has letters written on it. Pieces of paper have been bound around a few of the bones with leather thongs—these aren't just bones, they're relics. The skulls on the ledge haven't been labeled. They must have belonged to ordinary monks. I like to think those died peacefully of old age in their narrow beds.

The monk has turned his face away from the camera. Maybe he doesn't want to have his picture taken. Maybe he even considers it a sacrilege. It makes you wonder what the photographer had to do to get this picture. Who gave him permission? Did he even ask? He must have known a great picture when he saw one. Did he pose the monk against the skulls? Did he shoot a whole roll? Once you've taken the first picture, I know, it's easy to snap a second and a third. People will stand for it.

The monk has averted his face. Maybe, secretly, he is bloated with pride because he is the one who was chosen to display the bones, but I don't know—it seems to be a gesture of humility. Blank as the wall, he seems to be saying, I'm blank as the wall, stock-stone-still like the stone ledge holding the pile of skulls, holding out this box with the bones in it as proof—someone was here.

But fleetingly, you think—because *you* don't—maybe he just doesn't want to look into the box. Maybe he finds the bones disgusting.

Maybe not. Maybe he reveres them so, he has to avert his face, because they're so holy.

You glance back at the bones in the box. The skulls on the ledge are as clean as cattle skulls picked clean, sun-bleached in the desert. The bones in the box look mottled, rotted. Maybe not. Maybe they've been polished, varnished to a darker hue. One of the skulls has fallen forward and almost seems to be gnawing on the edge of the box.

Like the round "O" in the skull behind him, the black hole of the monk's convoluted ear seems somehow articulate. His unseen eyes are eloquent. When I opened the magazine in a waiting room and saw this photo, I was sure this man was signaling, he could hardly bear to show us what was in the box.

But someone, I thought, has to tend to the bones. Someone has to arrange and rearrange the display. Someone has to take the box down off the shelf to show you. This is that man.

1985

Happy are men who yet before they are killed
Can let their veins run cold.
Whom no compassion fleers
Or makes their feet
Sore on the alleys cobbled with their brothers.

—*Wilfred Owen*

GREENWICH VILLAGE, NEW YORK CITY

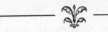

A tangle of streets, many of them still lined with low houses, this part of New York was once a true village, a remote suburb and resort from the plague that coursed through lower Manhattan in the early 19th century. Time was, dairy maids from New Jersey would row across the Hudson to sell their buttermilk in the Village, clam barges would tie up at the waterfront, and bloody beef would hang on hooks at the butchers' along the length of Washington Street.

Skirting quaint old Greenwich Village, the gridded city marched uptown. Because it remained a backwater and a low-rent refuge, the Village attracted artists and thinkers. By the 1920s, it had became internationally known as the cradle of American Bohemianism, teeming with noncon-formists, a hotbed of free love. Art, politics, and passion were inseparable from the romance of the Village, with its smoke-filled cafes, cobbled lanes, and unmade beds.

Not quite as notorious as the bottle parties and Bolshe-vik coffeehouses, one aspect of Village life was neverthe-less apparent to anyone who walked its streets open eyed: a certain kind of man and a certain kind of woman had staked a claim on the Village. In the popular mind, *he* was a narrow-shouldered figure retreating in haste down a shadowed alley, but *she* stood planted on the sidewalk, arms akimbo, fists on her hips.

In the summer of 1969, when a routine vice raid on a Village gay bar turned into a riot and the police were routed, the real people behind these stereotypes began to come to life in living color on TV, in the Sunday supplements, and on the glossy pages of national news magazines. What the formerly cowed college kids, hustlers, and drag queens at the Stonewall Inn were saying was, "This is ours, you can't close it down, you can't take it away." Soon gays—men and women alike—were mugging for the camera and shouting their names out loud. Gay liberation had begun.

New York's Greenwich Village had always been a powerful magnet for young gay men from all over the United States, but by the 1980s, there was an openly gay presence in the Village that far exceeded the fantasies of any 50s "homophile." The so-called gay lifestyle centered around bars ranged along the waterfront, up and down Christopher Street, tucked away on side streets. It throbbed in early-morning dance clubs and discos in lofts and garages. It embraced back-room sex bars in the meat-packing district. Professional associations, theatre groups, and political organizations were a part of gay life, but so were X-rated bookstores, Turkish baths, and porno movies. What local politicians were schooled to refer to as the "gay community" was a highly sexual entity—after all, wasn't this minority defined solely by its sexuality to begin with?

In the wake of gay liberation married men, bisexual men, and other putative nongays were, as always, a part of the gay world, but furtive sex no longer characterized it. Anonymous sex, however, did. In word, if not in deed, most if not all of the members of this new generation of self-defined gay men were militantly sexual. In reaction to past repression, they embraced promiscuity (but didn't call it that), rejected the middle-class ideal of monogamy, and promoted what Freud termed "polymorphous perversity." In this, they closely resembled their urban heterosexual peers, but being single males, they had more latitude—and maybe even more inclination—to act on their theories than most of their straight counterparts did.

The gay psychosocial/political program had its critics, right and left, who pointed out that it wasn't merely incidental that the word "clone" had been coined to describe the new gay man—rigid in demeanor, costumed in conformity, basically conservative, the gay ghetto-dweller gazed inward, not outward to society at large. This reality, however, didn't fit the image of enlightened and even unbridled hedonism that gays—particularly the commercial gay media, with its advertising base in the sex industry—wanted to promote.

Of course, here as in every city, there were gay couples leading thoroughly bourgeois lives, sharing property, cars, and houses with mortgages on them. Coupling was still a goal for lots of gay men. But finally, the venereal disease clinic was as central to this subculture as was the Oscar Wilde Memorial Bookshop.

Was it a lifestyle—which implied, of course, that gay identity could be taken up and sluffed off as easily as a pair of jeans—a culture, or a community? Clearly, it was a potent subculture that made vital contributions on many levels, especially through fashion and the fine and performing arts, to the life of New York and the nation. Until the historical accident that signaled the advent of AIDS, however, it couldn't be called a community.

1. THE PIRANHA

February 15, 1985. At 6:30 a.m., as on every weekday morning, the alarm rings and Dennis rolls out of bed. Soon Jim hears the sound of the shower.

Every morning when Jim wakes up, as soon as he opens his eyes, he asks himself, Am I going to get out of bed today? Am I going to bounce out of bed? Or am I going to lie here? Every morning he wakes up to that.

This apartment isn't big enough for two people. It's a ground-floor studio with a closetlike kitchen. A double platform bed and a sectional sofa take up a lot of the room. There is a big round coffee table with a mirrored top. There is a complete sound system in a cabinet with smoked Lucite doors. There is a bookcase and a large stereo speaker standing on top of an upright footlocker. There is a kitchen table with three chairs in front of the shuttered windows. There is too much—too much junk, too much furniture. Most of it came with the apartment. And Jim and Dennis both have things in storage besides— most of Jim's stuff is still in Houston.

Any decorative touches in the room are due to Dennis. The deer head above the little fireplace belongs to Dennis, as do the framed Erté prints on the opposite wall.

11

Dennis is a display director at a department store on Long Island. A vinyl satchel on the floor under the coffee table holds Dennis's knitting. Some books and an underlining pen lie on a cushion at the corner of the sofa where Dennis likes to sit. One of the books is *Risking*, by David Viscott, M.D. The cover says it will help you make crucial choices in your life.

A typewriter sits on the floor in the corner. A stack of magazines sits on the table—*National Geographic Traveler, Gourmet,* several copies of *Television/Radio Age.* Jim is a media buyer for a small agency. A cane with a decorative handle leans against the wall nearby. This was Jim's Valentine's Day present from Dennis yesterday.

Jim gets out of bed at 7:00. Dennis is out of the shower. Jim goes into the bathroom. The bathroom is tiny, so they've fallen into this routine.

By 7:30, Dennis is gone—he drives to his job. Jim sits down at the kitchen table with his cigarettes and a cup of coffee and gets down to work. Today is essentially his last day on the job. He's been working at home for the past six weeks. He's just putting the finishing touches on a big project. It's been frustrating, working out of the house and not being in the office, having to do everything over the phone and write endless memos because you can't just lean in the door and talk to someone. But he's proud of himself. This project would have been a monumental job for a well person to do.

The phone starts ringing at about 9. Jim's boss calls and they talk about the schedules Jim is finishing. In the middle of the conversation Jim says, "You know, I'm pissed at you."

"Why?"

"Because you brought in my replacement yesterday and you didn't tell me about it. I thought we had a better relationship than that."

"Jim, I'm really sorry. I've just been so busy."

They've been meaning to have lunch for weeks.

After he talks to his boss, Jim calls a friend, a woman at another agency where he used to work. Yesterday, when he felt especially crazy and pressured, she dropped by unannounced to cheer Jim up. Most of the friends he has in New York would never consider dropping by like that. In Texas, people were dropping by his house all the time. In New York you have to make an appointment to drop by.

He calls an acquaintance in L.A. with a question about syndicated programming. He calls Scott in Dallas to wish him a belated happy Valentine's Day and see how he's doing. Scott has spinal meningitis. Jim has never met Scott—a few months ago a friend in Texas asked Jim if he'd call Scott, who was alone and confused. Now they talk on the phone almost every day.

He calls Edward. Edward is Jim's counselor from the Gay Men's Health Crisis. Bitterly, Jim lays into his boss. "I ought to spit in the back of someone's throat." Jim talks this way when he's mad, which is most of the time.

"Why are you so upset?" Edward asks after a while.

Because it's his last day at work, because he will probably never work again unless there is a cure for what he has, because he is no longer of use. But Jim says, "They did it without letting me know."

"What did he say?"

"He forgot to tell me."

Jim puts on a light jacket and goes out to the corner grocery for cigarettes. The people who run the grocery are Asian. They don't speak much English so there is a lot of playacting—How are you today, fine, good, yes yes yes. Jim's a regular customer. Before he got sick, he'd walk in and they'd take down a pack of Winstons automatically. He never had to ask. Then he went to Merit Ultra-Lights. They'd still reach for the Winstons and he'd have to say no no no. And now he smokes Carltons.

Back home, Jim finishes his project. Then he strips the bed and takes a load of laundry down to the basement.

He comes back upstairs and sweeps the floor, fixes a sandwich, pours another cup of coffee.

He eats lunch sitting next to the windows. It's sunny. The shutters are open. People pass by. Gay-boys pass by in bomber jackets and jeans. Old women and winos pass by. Trucks rumble by. The oil man comes. Maybe once a week, the oil man pulls up and runs a hose to the hookup in the sidewalk. Sometimes the faces are familiar, and Jim waves.

Since he began working at home, Jim has gotten friendly with other people in the building. There's one woman with a little boy—they laugh and joke. A few days ago, Jim ran into them out in the hall at the mailboxes. It was snowing out. "Are you taking this poor child out in that wicked weather?" Jim asked the woman.

"Wicked weather, Mama, wicked weather!" Little kids catch on so fast.

Jim goes down and puts the clothes in the drier, putters around the apartment, picks things up, straightens up, takes the clothes out of the drier, puts in another load. The phone rings. It's Frank, the office messenger. He's coming down. Frank's been shuttling back and forth since Jim started working at home. Frank's going to bring Jim's paycheck. Jim needs that check.

One night recently, Jim Sharp and Edward Dunn spent a few hours together discussing God, mortality, and eternity. Edward, who has pronounced opinions on most subjects, says he has no answers on this one. Lately, he says, he's been asking more questions. Jim, born and raised in Texas and a regular churchgoer, will tell you tongue in cheek that his idea of heaven "based on my childhood beliefs" is "a canasta game with lots of coffee and cigarettes." But he's been asking more questions, too. He's concluded, he says, that God will not give him more than he can handle.

Officially, Edward is Jim's "crisis intervention worker,"

a counselor from the Gay Men's Health Crisis, which
provides outpatient assistance to New Yorkers with AIDS
like Jim. Edward's job is to help Jim and his lover Dennis
through the many difficulties—financial, legal, medical—
they're certain to encounter due to Jim's condition. Jim
has had one of the opportunistic infections that indicate
severe immune deficiency but it was a relatively light case.
He hasn't yet had anything else major so there have been
no repeated, protracted hospital stays. If they come, Edward is ready for them. He knows about AIDS. His own
lover died of it less than 18 months ago.

After a rocky beginning last fall, Jim and Edward became friends. "In this job," Edward says, "you have to
maintain a lot of distance. He adds wryly, "It says here in
fine print." In fact, his relationship with Jim has grown
into one of special intensity. "We're not talking here about
visiting the sick and reading to them. It's certainly one of
the most intimate relationships I will ever have. I see
Jim—and that could be me there. It's a mirror. It's not a
victim-savior relationship. We're the same person. We're
just on different sides of the fence."

Nevertheless, there is a certain artfully maintained distance between them. Until recently, Jim hadn't even introduced Edward to Dennis, maybe because to do so would
have made AIDS more irrevocably real—or as Edward
puts it, "bring AIDS into his home." And Jim doesn't
know very much about Edward's late lover, Robert. Once
when he asked about Robert's death, the sadness in Edward's eyes was so profound, Jim knew not to ask again.

Jim and Edward are both aggressive go-getters. They
share many common interests and the same caustic sense
of humor. If they'd met under different circumstances,
they agree, they would have become friends. But ulti-
mately, however friendly they might be, Jim and Edward
are both aware that Edward isn't really there to be Jim's
friend. He's there to help Jim live with AIDS. Now, after

months of fear, rage, and denial, Jim is willing to try to do that.

On top of a stereo speaker in Jim's apartment is a stuffed piranha. Edward brought it back from Brazil last winter and when he gave it to Jim he said, joking, "This is how you look when you don't get your way."

The fish is mounted as if poised for attack, bristling, jaws agape. Like AIDS, the piranha is at first glance shocking, repulsive. But on closer inspection, it doesn't look real. It looks like something whipped up out of latex and horsehair for some low-budget horror movie. Thus demystified, it can be dismissed—that is, until your eye happens to fall on it again. Then you wish it weren't in the same room with you.

AIDS won't go away. Four years into the epidemic, it is now a fact of life for thousands upon thousands of Americans—even if most of them don't yet know it.

Last year, three years after the first indications of this mysterious breakdown of the immune system were discovered in Los Angeles, San Francisco, and New York, scientists announced the discovery of a virus they believed caused it. Called by the Americans HTLV-III and by the French LAV,* this "retrovirus" literally turns cells around, counter to their usual purposes. It invades white blood cells called T-helper cells, the very cells meant to defend the body against outside infections. Once inside the T-cell, the virus may lay dormant for years before utilizing the genetic material of the cell to crank out copies of the virus.

AIDS is almost always fatal. Most people with AIDS die within 18 months after diagnosis. The mortality rate for AIDS has been established at 95–100 percent two years after onset.

---

*Later, the virus was universally called HIV, for Human Immunodeficiency Virus. Soon after its discovery, AIDS itself was for a while called GRID, for Gay-Related Immunodeficiency.

Initially, the AIDS story was reported vigorously in the gay press and almost not at all in the general media. But public concern over the disease suddenly burgeoned in 1983 and something very close to panic gripped parts of the country.

The piranha thrives on terror. Acts of violence against gay men—or those perceived to be gay men—increased. Funeral homes refused to bury the AIDS dead. Stories already abounded about hospital workers so frightened of the disease that they left food trays outside rooms and refused AIDS patients the most elementary amenities. Now discrimination against people with AIDS or those perceived to have AIDS became relatively common. Some people with AIDS—or suspected of having AIDS, even suspected of associating with people with AIDS—were ostracized on the job or fired outright. They were evicted from their apartments. Often they were abandoned by friends and acquaintances, by loved ones as well.

When the discovery of the so-called AIDS virus was announced, it helped to quiet fears but it also engendered what amounts to a false complacency among the general public, which seems content to believe that somehow the epidemic has been contained.

The number of those stricken by AIDS continues to double every six months. No cure is in sight and a vaccine, if it can be developed, is probably years away. Moreover, researchers are discovering, upwards of one million Americans have already been exposed to the virus. AIDS is widespread in parts of Africa. Worldwide, many more thousands of people than scientists initially forecasted will certainly die in the next decade of the opportunistic diseases that accompany immune deficiency. What might have been viewed just a few years ago as something of a medical curiosity has erupted into a large-scale human catastrophe with international dimensions. AIDS can no longer be ignored.

AIDS is not and never has been "a gay disease." To

moderate their hereditary bleeding condition, hemophiliacs use a product known as Factor VIII, which is concentrated from the blood of as many as 20,000 donors. A number of hemophiliacs who use Factor VIII have contracted the AIDS virus from it. Thus far, 100 cases of AIDS have been reported among hemophiliacs or those who received tainted transfusions before the virus was discovered in the blood supply and methods were instituted to screen it out. In 1985, intravenous drug abusers, who acquire the virus if they share contaminated needles, comprise 17 percent of AIDS cases nationwide.

Scientists now think AIDS initially manifested itself in this country around 1979. It was first noticed, however, a few years later in gay men, who had come into contact with the virus during sex. The blood of sexually active gay men was remarkably conducive to the spread of AIDS. Many young gay men had serial, anonymous sexual partners and were already at risk for other infectious diseases like hepatitis. Anal intercourse, in particular, offers a ready avenue into the bloodstream.

In 1981, the number of diagnosed AIDS cases in the United States hovered at 100. One year later the total had climbed to over 300. By the summer of 1983, there were nearly 1,500 cases. This week—in the middle of February 1985—the official count of people with AIDS in America stands at 8,495. Of those, 6,136 are homosexual males—73 percent of the total.*

As it was in the beginning and remains, most of the dead in the foreseeable future will be homosexual men. Thus, the onus of the AIDS epidemic will continue to fall on the increasingly besieged gay community, which in

*By February 1987, two years later, AIDS cases in the U.S. had more than tripled. Gay men accounted for 66 percent of those diagnosed (or 20,094), intravenous drug users, 17 percent (or 5,155). Over the course of time, there were gradual and steady increases in the percentages of women and children diagnosed.

most cities has shouldered primary responsibility for crucial counseling, public information, and support services.

In New York, the nonprofit Gay Men's Health Crisis, through volunteers like Edward, almost singlehandedly provides nonmedical outpatient assistance to fully 42 percent of the people with AIDS in the city. One indication of how much New York City relies on GMHC is that all callers to the health department who request AIDS-related social services are referred to GMHC. The organization is clocking 100 new clients a month. Its caseload has quadrupled in the past year.

GMHC volunteers—"buddies," counselors, advisers—carry out tasks that range from grocery shopping to in-hospital patient advocacy to unraveling the endless financial and legal complications the disease entails. Those services are provided free of charge and without regard to sexual preference. In fact, two out of five people served by GMHC are heterosexual.

Since the epidemic began, most of the money raised to counsel New Yorkers with AIDS has come from the gay community alone—in the form of donations to GMHC, the nascent American Foundation for AIDS Research, and the AIDS Resource Center, which works to provide housing for people with AIDS. But private-sector funding is no longer equal to the task.

Prodded by a few persistent members of Congress, the federal government has recently pumped research money for AIDS into the budget, but federal funds for outpatient social services are virtually nonexistent. Allocations from governments in states where AIDS is currently most prevalent vary. New York State has formed an AIDS Institute which distributes funds almost exclusively earmarked for research and education. New York State monies currently make up 25 percent of GMHC's annual budget.

With over 3,000 cases and reporting three to four new

cases of AIDS each day, New York City is at the epicenter of the epidemic, yet during the last fiscal year, the city government allocated only $41,000 to GMHC, its primary outpatient provider. This is compared to San Francisco's allocation of $1.5 million for comparable private-sector efforts—to serve one third the cases. In per capita terms, as of January 7 this year, San Francisco was spending $1,595.32 in social service support funds on each person with AIDS, while New York City was spending $14.75.

The poor record of the Koch administration in relation to AIDS has made it a target of angry allegations and the mayor, a longtime advocate of gay rights, has lost the support of many gay men and lesbians who feel the city is paying too little attention to the epidemic too late.

Given its limited financial resources and the spiraling AIDS caseload, says Roger McFarlane, GMHC's executive director, the organization has reached the limit of the number of people it can serve. Human resources, he points out, are abundant—qualified, dedicated volunteers have been plentiful since GMHC was founded three years ago by a handful of concerned men, and "that's irreplace-able, you could never pay for that."

Among gay men and women nationwide, AIDS has led to acts of remarkable altruism, even heroism. Just one example—lesbians in San Diego have formed an organization called Blood Sisters to make up for a shortfall in the blood supply due to the voluntary withdrawal of gay male donors.

"We've done things we would never have thought we would be called upon to do in the context of community," says Virginia Apuzzo, until recently executive director of the New York-based National Gay and Lesbian Task Force. "We've visited the sick and buried the dead. And we did it not just because it had to be done, but also because nobody else would do it."

AIDS has politicized many for whom the left-leaning gay rights movement of the early 1970s seemed remote.

It has brought about for others a reevaluation of personal and spiritual priorities. What is just being grasped now is the extent to which AIDS has also traumatized a generation—Edward's and Jim's generation—of vital young men, in their thirties and forties, who once might have scanned the personal advertisements in their local gay newspapers, for diversion if not for partners, and now dread the inevitable obituaries.

2. MY LIFE CHANGED

There's a roll of film Edward Dunn can't bring himself to develop. On it is a photograph of him and his lover Robert, taken by a nurse at New York Hospital in November 1983. Edward says echoes are forming around memories that used to be crisp. There is a kind of separation happening, he says. But he still has a recollection of what Robert looked like when the photo was taken, a month or so before his death.

Watching Robert die from AIDS was, says Edward, like standing by powerless while a freight train roared through his life. Last July, when he called GMHC to volunteer, he did it because "I felt desperately that I had to be doing something. I couldn't just sit by impotently and watch." He wanted to make a difference. He hadn't, he felt, made enough of a difference for Robert.

There was another reason for volunteering. As anyone intimately acquainted with AIDS will tell you, once you've seen it, you are never the same. Most of Edward's friends, caught up in their own fears, avoided even talking about AIDS. Edward says he needed to know "that somebody else knew what I knew." His GMHC counseling team is composed of people who do. Among them is a young

23

woman who came to New York from the Midwest to help nurse her brother, who was dying of AIDS, and found herself so altered by the experience of his death that she couldn't go back home.

At GMHC, they suggested Edward do what they called crisis intervention counseling. They warned him that it can be horrendous work. But Edward wasn't afraid. What could possibly be worse than watching the human being you loved most in the world die from AIDS?

In the training sessions, Edward listened to other new volunteers talk about death and AIDS. They talked about AIDS, it occurred to him, as if it were a kind of gentle, Camille-like wasting away. But Edward knew—he'd seen— AIDS is about shit and blood.

In August of last year, Edward received his first assignment. He went to the GMHC offices and read the intake report on Jim Sharp, who had just been diagnosed with a syndrome commonly called AIDS-Related Complex, or ARC.

As scientists have come to understand, AIDS is not a black-and-white illness but a spectrum of immune deficiency. Characterized especially by swollen lymph nodes and persistent fever, ARC is sometimes called "pre-AIDS" by doctors since it falls short of a complete suppression of the immune system.

It's now thought that for every person infected with the AIDS virus who goes on to develop full-blown AIDS, there are ten with ARC. Sometimes ARC turns into AIDS, sometimes it doesn't. Estimates vary on the percentage of cases where it does. Researchers estimate that from 4 to 19 percent of people infected with the virus will eventually develop AIDS.*

In Jim's case, ARC turned into AIDS in December,

---

*Since 1985, most AIDS experts have revised this estimate and now believe that from 20 percent to 30 percent of HIV-infected people will develop AIDS symptoms within five years of exposure to the virus. Current medical thinking is that virtually every HIV-infected person will eventually manifest AIDS.

when his doctor made an empirical diagnosis of *pneumocystis carinii* pneumonia—"empirical" because he didn't insist on a confirmatory lung biopsy and simply gave Jim medication that seemed to clear up this rare lung infection. *Pneumocystis* is one of the two diseases physicians first noticed in gay men and connected with immune suppression in 1981. Since then, the Centers for Disease Control in Atlanta has used *pneumocystis* and Kaposi's sarcoma, a highly unusual skin cancer, to define AIDS.

"The whole thing to me is AIDS," says Jim's lover Dennis. "As far as I'm concerned, from day one it was AIDS." And all Jim himself knew last August was that he'd been abruptly jettisoned out of the legions of the "worried well" and into the ranks of the "walking wounded."

Some people fall to pieces when they receive the kind of news Jim had. But, Edward recalls, at their first meeting in Jim's apartment, Jim appeared quite calm.

There had been an attempt at GMHC to match them. Jim learned that Edward was a freelance advertising copy-writer. Edward already knew Jim had left a good job in advertising in Houston the year before and took a substantial salary cut to come to New York because he felt he had to challenge the citadel of the business. He'd done well.

Jim asked Edward if he'd like a cup of coffee. Stiffly, formally, they chatted for an hour or so. Edward offered his services but, curiously, they didn't talk directly about AIDS. Edward remembers, it was "as if there were a dead elephant in the middle of the floor and we were both too polite to mention it."

Edward was nervous. A man with a terminal illness sat opposite him but he didn't know how willing Jim was to discuss it. It was only a few weeks after the training, a two-day marathon that had nevertheless left him, it seemed, unequipped to talk about AIDS with this man—his first, his very first client. He was convinced he wasn't up to the job. He was peering into the future. Would he be able to help this polite stranger through the labyrinth Robert had entered two years before?

Jim smoked cigarette after cigarette—clearly, he had no intention of quitting smoking—but generally, Edward thought, for a man who was facing a condition most people regarded as a death sentence, Jim seemed almost blasé.

Jim was most assuredly not blasé. He was terrified. He knew what AIDS meant. He knew what happens. Your friends desert you, your lover kicks you out onto the street. You get fired, you get evicted from your apartment. You're a leper. You die alone.

The day the doctor told Jim, he walked out of the office onto Central Park West and down the sidewalk in a daze. It was a beautiful day. All he could think was, This isn't funny. It was as if God had been lounging around up there with the angels and had just decided,

Now, let's give it to—hmmm—Jim Sharp!

This is not funny, Jim thought. After all the other crap that's gone down in my life, this isn't funny.

Things were going great. He'd only been in New York a year and a half and he'd found a job he loved and the lover he'd always dreamed of. Then in one visit to the doctor, everything got turned inside out.

"My life changed. My life changed. You walk into some doctor's office and he tells you you have the beginnings of a disease no one has an answer for, that you've been reading about in the newspaper, that is killing people, that you've just had a friend die of." Jim pauses. "I very much like being in control. The control was taken away. I was relieved because I finally knew what was going on inside of me—but it was sort of like waiting for the Germans to attack at the Battle of the Bulge? You're sick and tired of waiting for the attack to come, but when it does, you're not really relieved because there are bullets whizzing around your head. It's a 'Catch-22' situation."

The doctor encouraged Jim to continue working, not to drop out and go onto disability as some people were.

"I most certainly will continue working."

He walked out onto the street.

Jim called GMHC because he knew he'd need help. Now he was meeting a so-called "crisis intervention worker." But it was like watching someone else go through the motions. Jim knew he was really in this alone.

Jim grew up poor. He put himself through school and forged ahead mainly on the currency of his own considerable native intelligence. A recovered alcoholic, Jim had saved his life once before. If sheer willpower meant anything, Jim would save his life again.

Feeling disoriented soon after he moved to New York, Jim had sought out a psychotherapist. Jim's therapist says Jim "has this image of himself as a cowboy, a person who can pull himself together" no matter what. Jim agrees. He says he grew up to believe "that you get up in the morning and you pull your boots on by the straps. You get up and go.

"This disease has taught me," he adds in his soft drawl, "that this is not necessarily so."

3. THE FOOT IN THE DOOR

Jim's sole request of Edward that first month was that he help him find a dentist, so Edward gave him the name of one registered at GMHC as willing to treat people with AIDS. Jim also allowed Edward to enroll him in a support group at GMHC for people with AIDS, but at the meeting he got into an argument with the group leader, who said he couldn't smoke. Jim smoked anyway. He did not go back. The truth was, Jim identified with the sickest man in the room and it scared him to death.

He still looked good. On the street he would see people with AIDS—he knew enough about the symptoms to notice the swollen nodes in the neck. It made him sad. He felt sorry for those men. But now his own body was telling him, You have it too.

Edward called regularly. Jim was distant. No, his lover didn't need a support group—anyway, Dennis was too busy at work. Jim was feeling fine. Everything was fine. Jim presented the same bland, good ol' boy facade to Edward he was adept at projecting in business.

"Jim can put up a wonderful front," Edward says. "Very breezy. He can be charming and light. Evasive."

Gradually, Edward began to understand. He was on

the outside and Jim wasn't going to let him in. Jim had
his life strictly compartmentalized—his lover, his therapist, his doctor, his job. It was as if Jim were in a room
with four doors. Every once in a while he'd open one of
them, but for the most part he remained alone in the
center, isolated.

In addition, Edward began to understand the essence
of the crisis Jim was enduring. Jim was in crisis precisely
to the degree that he needed to deny that any crisis
existed.

Edward saw he quite literally represented AIDS to Jim.
And Jim was determined—maybe AIDS had its foot in
the door, but he was damned if he would let it into the
house.

He was deluded. AIDS had moved in.

Jim's response to AIDS was far from atypical. AIDS, it
often seems, is as much about denial as it is about death.
*I don't really have it. I won't let it stop me. I'm going to beat
it.* Denial is a powerful, often healthy, initial reaction. In
the face of an AIDS diagnosis, short-term, even total
denial can be the only thing that wards off a nervous breakdown. Being able to say, *I know I have it but who knows what
that means?* can be what's called a *mitzvah* in Yiddish, a
godsend. Continuing denial of one aspect or another of
the disease can be a way of protecting oneself from the
unremitting fears that accompany it. *It's not going to happen to me that way* is a means to assert one's individuality
in the midst of an ego-leveling calamity. Denial explains
why the person who has been diagnosed often seems
utterly immune to the consequences of the disease. Family and friends might be devastated, but he or she seems
to reside in the calm center of the eye of the storm. And
it shouldn't be forgotten that *I'm different* is quite literally
true—each case *is* different, bringing with it its own set of
circumstances.

Accepting the reality of a terminal disease—a reality

that is often shrouded and complicated, slow to reveal itself—is a wrenching process. Some never fully accept. Edward's lover Robert, for instance, wasn't ever able to accept the full implications of having AIDS. At the end, Edward needed to say good-bye to Robert and tell him how much he'd miss him. But Robert, even in the last excruciating months of his illness, couldn't admit he was dying.

Loved ones of the afflicted can promote elaborate denial. Parents often learn simultaneously about AIDS and a son's homosexuality—or his drug abuse. Sometimes they choose not to deal with the existence of either. And although hospice workers are struck by the breadth of support gay men can summon up from friends and lovers, peers sometimes postpone coming to terms with the role AIDS plays in their own lives by avoiding friends who have it.

Dixie Beckham, a psychotherapist in private practice who also runs a support group at GMHC for people with AIDS, notes the severe isolation they experience. "There are so many taboos a gay man who is dying of AIDS has to deal with," she says, "it would be easier to talk about an amputation." And, of course, there is still unwarranted fear of contagion. Most people would not so much as touch an AIDS patient. Even now when so much more is known about its transmission, AIDS continues to carry with it wholly inappropriate associations of a contagious plague, rather than an infectious disease.

There is a particularly cruel dimension to AIDS. The piranha not only churns up terror, it swims in a medium charged with shame and guilt. At its most rudimentary, "AIDS denial" reflects the tacit judgment of society that AIDS happens only to an outcast few—people who somehow deserve the disease. Jim says he and his lover Dennis paid little attention to AIDS until he was diagnosed. It was not something that happened to churchgoing people like them who were in a monogamous relationship.

Daniel William, a New York City physician whose practice is largely composed of homosexual men, says the misconception—shared by gays and heterosexuals alike—that only "fast-trackers" with phenomenal numbers of sexual contacts get AIDS is a continuing "travesty." Many of the men first diagnosed with AIDS did report that they'd had up to twice as many anonymous sexual encounters as others in control studies. Recently, however, says Dr. William, he has been diagnosing AIDS in men "whose sexual lives were, I think, probably on a par with many single women in Manhattan—they dated and had serial monogamy. They had one person in their life at a time." It is now simply far easier for a gay or bisexual man to come into contact with the AIDS virus. In fact, it's so widespread, says James Curran, head of the AIDS section at the Centers for Disease Control, a "single sexual contact for a gay man in New York or San Francisco, or many other American cities, now means a substantial risk of getting infected."

As markedly lower rates of sexually transmitted diseases among gay men attest, most who are sexually active have radically altered their behavior in response to the epidemic. Many have simply chosen to be chaste. Yet the ongoing dread and uncertainty surrounding AIDS, it seems, has not prevented a large segment of the gay population—one third in a San Francisco survey last year—from continuing or resuming high-risk sexual activity. On the contrary, the fact that dread and uncertainty *are* ongoing might be discouraging many from avoiding exposure to the virus.

AIDS denial in sexually active gay and bisexual men can prevent early diagnosis of the condition, hamper treatment of the diseases that accompany AIDS, encourage illusions of immunity.

Jim Graham, executive director of the community-based Whitman-Walker Clinic in Washington, D.C., feels many gay men there have come to view AIDS "as a crap shoot—

something that happens in a thoroughly serendipitous way."
Stephen F. Morin, a San Francisco psychologist studying
gay men in that city, notes that many continue to maintain the erroneous "conviction that they have been exposed to the virus and have successfully fought it off."
Jim's psychotherapist, who sees as many gay as heterosexual clients, says some of them seem to employ "a filter
merchanism" regarding AIDS—"It's just not happening."
New York City Health Commissioner David Sencer has
noted that education for prevention has thus far been
"based on fear, and preliminary data indicate that the
fear may be wearing off."

AIDS is an incurable disease, so its prevention through
education is crucial, but there are indications that denial
on the part of risk-taking men is being encouraged by the
inability or failure of some segments of the public health
establishment to deliver adequate and concise information on prevention. Most sexually active gay men have
received the message via the gay media that they are to
engage in "safe sex." The definition of safe sex being
published in gay magazines, newspapers, and newsletters
has not been drawn up by government scientists but by a
national association of gay physicians who do not themselves pretend to know absolutely what safe sex—beyond
no sex at all—is. So phrases like "less risky" and euphemisms like "no exchange of bodily fluids" must take the
place of confident prohibitions against, say, oral intercourse and kissing. The list of "maybes" is a long one.
And in the meantime, to date no one at the Centers for
Disease Control has bothered to study the efficacy of
condoms as a barrier against the virus.

The general public might well be learning that AIDS
cannot be transmitted through casual contact, but there
are thousands of people in risk groups who do not know
how, why, or even that they are at risk. The GMHC
hotline receives 2,000 calls per month from such people.
In New York City, in 1985, with over a third of the cases

in the United States, there are still no pamphlets on AIDS prevention in city-run venereal disease clinics.

If AIDS denial extends to politicians and civil servants, why should physicians and other health-care workers be exempt? After all, they're on the front lines of the epidemic. Is it any wonder that there are doctors reluctant to count—and even to report—newly diagnosed AIDS cases in their practices? One Manhattan internist who has lost dozens of patients confesses that one of his most persistent fears is that he might not spot early symptoms of AIDS in patients he's known for a long time and feels particularly close to.

Denial does not stop with death. Edward found, when Robert died, that society has not "necessarily dictated how you should react when your gay son loses his lover to a horrifying, deadly, possibly disreputable disease." His attempts to discuss his loss with his family were deflected, as if nothing had happened.

"Hi, Jim. How are you feeling?"

"Oh, I'm feeling fine."

"You're not at work today. Why didn't you go to work today?"

"Oh, because I woke up and I was real tired."

"So are you really feeling fine?"

"Well, I'm not really feeling fine."

As winter approached, Jim started getting colds he couldn't shake, bouts of flu. He was experiencing chronic and worsening exhaustion. Every week, it seemed, there was another hitch, another irritation—a fungus in his throat, night sweats, aches. Still, and in spite of his doctor's warnings, Jim continued to work long hours and take on more projects. When Edward called, he stonewalled.

"I had a very difficult time trusting him," Jim says. "He was dealing with a very intimate part of my life that I didn't want to acknowledge. If he was around, I had to acknowledge it."

Trying to help Jim at that time was, says Edward, "like hard-rock mining—time-consuming, minute work. I would have to keep at him to get him to admit there was anything wrong at all." Not infrequently, instead of saying good-bye when they had finished talking on the phone, Jim would abruptly hang up.

"It left me hanging there," Edward says. "I really think he was testing me to see how much I was going to put up with. He was getting really feisty—a little hostile. I would call him up and he would be nonresponsive—like he couldn't care less whether he was talking to me or not. Not what he would say, just his attitude, lack of interest. I would see him and he would pitch his voice—Jim has a very deep voice—he would pitch it in such a way that I couldn't understand what he was saying. He would really make me work. I think he wanted to see if I was really going to be there. He was getting more scared.

"The first time he pissed me off, I immediately thought, Oh God, I can't be pissed off, this person has a fatal disease. That point of view serves no one. No one.

"I wasn't scared of him but I was scared of what he represented. I was afraid of the challenge—because I hadn't been able to do anything for my lover. I hadn't been able to make everything okay. With Jim, I didn't want to make any mistakes."

After Jim's ARC diagnosis, near the end of August, another blow came with the news that Dennis's father was dying in the Midwest. Dennis was gone for two weeks. Jim spent them alone. He went to work. He came home from work and watched TV. He was lethargic. He didn't want to talk to anyone. He was hurt that he couldn't be with Dennis. When Dennis' father died, Jim wasn't invited to the funeral. He remained depressed and immobilized. He told Edward things were fine.

But Jim was growing more angry. He was growing furious. He felt AIDS taking over. Things were slipping.

The further they slipped, the angrier Jim got—the more angry, the more out of control—the more out of control, the more frightened. Fear and rage pinwheeled in him.

AIDS was taking over. Every conversation—with his lover, his friends, even with people who didn't know—was somehow tempered with it. Every phone call he got, it seemed, someone else had it.

He found himself wanting to knock people down in the street, innocent people, walking by, minding their own business. The simple fact that he had AIDS and they did not and they were blissfully going about their business untouched by AIDS infuriated him. Their ignorance, their immunity infuriated him. He still looked good. He was still walking around. They didn't have a clue as to what he—Jim Sharp—was going through. No one knew what he was in danger of losing. He didn't want to have AIDS. He wanted things to go on the way they were but they were not going to now. He was 34. It was not time for this to happen. No one cared. Just keep your mouth shut, Jim Sharp. Go about your business. No one knew and as long as he kept his mouth shut no one had to know—he was sinking, he was sad, he was hurting.

Jim spent whole days consumed with fury. During one visit he found himself shouting at his doctor—"All my life I've been going to the doctor's with a virus and they give me pills or a shot and I go home and I'm better in three days! Why can't you do this for me!"

Tough and aggressive on the outside, on the inside soft and generous to a fault, Jim had turned into a fury. When Edward gave him the piranha, both of them are well aware, it was not entirely a joke.

Edward expected hostility from Jim—GMHC workers are often used as targets for the unappeasable anger of people they're trying to help. Yet Jim didn't attack Edward directly. Instead, he feigned indifference, froze him out.

But not completely. Jim knew he couldn't afford to lose

Edward. To him Edward was a kind of spectral "step-father—he's here, he's going to help you, he'll pay the rent, and you have to put up with him."

The first test of this unacknowledged adoption came in October, when Jim's doctor decided to admit him to Cabrini Medical Center in Manhattan. Jim was constantly running a fever and his doctor wanted to make sure the cause of his swollen glands wasn't lymphatic cancer.

Edward and Jim talked often throughout the days Jim waited for a bed. Jim was very anxious. Edward rightly suspected that his denial regarding AIDS was "shredding" —cancer or not, Jim could no longer so successfully ignore the fact he was ill.

Edward was anxious, too. From his own experience, he knew "one thing always led to another." He and Jim seemed to be setting out on a path he'd trod with Robert two years before.

Jim says he went into the hospital "sort of hoping, wishing I had cancer—because if I had cancer, maybe I wouldn't have AIDS." But the first question the resident asked him was, "Are you a homosexual?"

"What?"

"Are you a homosexual?"

"Why?"

Because he had swollen glands. He fit the profile. But it shook him. He was only in for tests and they were already treating him like a person with AIDS.

After a few hitches, Jim got settled into his room. Around 6, Edward called. Jim realized he hadn't bothered to tell Edward he'd finally gone into the hospital, let alone his room number. And here was Edward—kind, patient Edward, who'd been putting out for months and getting nothing back—screaming at him on the phone.

"I've been calling the damned switchboard all afternoon trying to find you," Edward shouted into the receiver. "I called your doctor and they couldn't find you, nobody could find you. Why didn't you call me, for God's sake? I thought maybe you didn't go in, maybe you changed your mind—why the hell didn't you call me?"

Jim was stunned. He listened to Edward, mumbled a few words of apology, and hung up.

At home, Edward held his head in his hands. He knew he'd just destroyed any chance he'd ever had to help Jim.

Yet when Edward visited Jim the next day, he was friendly, even warm. "And he started doing something he hadn't done before. He started bitching about things— how terrible the food was and so forth. I thought I'd blown it, but I realized that day, I could be myself with this guy."

"I guess," says Jim, "I just finally got hit in the face— Edward's a human being, too, and he really cares about me."

4. HELL AND HIGH WATER

Jim's roommate in the hospital was a schoolteacher from Long Island, a family man, in for a liver test. He didn't know he was in the room with someone with AIDS—but then, Jim hadn't realized he was someone with AIDS, not really, not yet.

Jim affected a lack of concern about his upcoming surgery, but it scared him. He didn't like being in the hospital. He felt imprisoned. He didn't like taking orders. "I will do anything you ask me, anything—but don't tell me."

Jim had a violent reaction to the nuclear medicine test, where they put dye into your system. It kept him in the hospital a few extra days. They removed some glands from his neck and groin. When Jim lay sick in bed, his roommate answered his phone. They became friends.

Flowers kept arriving. Friends kept calling. Dennis went to work early so he could visit at the end of the day. Edward dropped by. Jim saw that a lot of people cared about him.

The hospital wore Jim out. By the time he left, he knew he had AIDS. He knew it was serious. Now he knew he had it. But he was back at work the next day.

No one seemed to be able to do anything about the fact that Jim's denial was making him more ill. One frigid day, his therapist ran into Jim on the street. Jim wasn't wearing a jacket. "Jim, why are you doing this to yourself? You're making yourself sick."

"He was working like a dog," Jim's doctor says. "This would become a major focus of our attention. Jim isn't unusual or atypical. He couldn't admit he was sick. We discussed this quite freely. I couldn't do anything. I could reinforce my feelings—don't push it until seven when your body feels like quitting at four." But Jim had never been a quitter.

One afternoon in October, Jim and Edward met for lunch at Mary Elizabeth's, a genteel cafe on East 37th Street. Jim and Edward were surrounded by ladies who lunch.

A sea change had taken place. Lately, when Edward asked Jim how things were going, he got the truth—some days it was all Jim could do to drag himself up the subway steps.

Jim looked good. He'd had an important meeting that day and was wearing a suit. Today Jim was feeling good. Edward was the one who felt rotten.

Jim's tests had turned out negative—no cancer. He was therefore "stable." People with AIDS need varying levels of support at various times. At Edward's last team meeting, the group leader turned to him and said, "Well, it looks like Jim Sharp is doing fine now. I think you can phase out so we can give you another client." Jim no longer needed a crisis worker. Edward knew the policy. He knew trained personnel were scarce. But he somehow felt this was wrong.

Edward felt that he'd made a contract with Jim and now he was being asked to betray him. It had always been in the back of Edward's mind that he was going to go through thick and thin with Jim, through hell and high water. Maybe it was naive and corny, but he'd all but promised that to Jim. What's more, he'd promised it to himself. He was going to see this through.

Edward thought it over. Maybe they know more about this than I do, he thought. Maybe this is what Jim needs right now, to feel independent. Maybe it will be a good thing for him. Maybe he'll even be flattered to see how well he's doing.

Yet he couldn't shake the feeling that what he was about to do was wrong. He waited until they'd finished eating. Jim leaned back and lit up a cigarette.

"Well, Jim," Edward began, "I think you're going to be doing fine by yourself now. You're doing so well, you don't need me anymore," Edward explained, "so technically our professional relationship is about to come to an end."

Jim sat bolt upright. His face flushed red. As Edward continued, Jim looked down at what was left of his lunch, up at the ceiling, anywhere but at Edward.

"Of course, I'll be in touch with you because—I mean, I care about your condition."

Jim put out his cigarette and immediately lit another. Sitting there amidst all the ladies lunching on Welsh rarebit, Jim wanted to rip Edward's face off.

"We'll continue to talk." Edward wondered if Jim would ever trust him again.

No, Jim thought, no. Edward couldn't leave. Edward was his ace in the hole. Edward was assigned to him. Edward had to put up with him no matter what. Anyone else could take a walk. Edward had to stay.

After months of trying to get rid of him, Jim heard himself saying to this familiar stranger, "I don't want you to go away."

Then after a moment, he heard Edward say, "Okay. Don't worry. I'll see what I can do."

Edward managed to stay on the case. A little more than a month later, Jim was diagnosed with *pneumocystis* pneumonia. That was conclusive evidence. Now he really had AIDS.

5. PERFECT BLOOD

On Labor Day weekend 1983, Edward took his lover Robert in an ambulance to New York Hospital. That same weekend Jim and Dennis met and fell in love.

The day after they met and exchanged phone numbers, Jim called Dennis. "See? I'm not one of those people who take your number and never call," Jim said. They made a date for the next week. They've seldom spent a night apart since.

"He would meet me after work," Dennis says. "I was taking the train home so he'd be at Penn Station every night at 9 o'clock when I got off the train. We'd go out to dinner or something and spend the night together."

Two months after they met and fell in love, Jim and Dennis found an apartment and moved in together. They didn't have to discuss whether or not they were lovers, Dennis explains—because they were lovers right from the beginning.

"We moved in together," Dennis says. "He fit into my family. All my friends liked him. It was like we'd been together forever. It was just this natural progression."

That Christmas they solemnized their relationship by exchanging rings. Now Jim's ring will fit over his index finger.

"I felt it would just go on forever," Dennis says. "We would work hard, maybe buy a house together somewhere someday, go on wonderful vacations, retire together somewhere—all the natural things people think about when they get into a relationship. I felt I was ready for a 'forever' relationship."

Last August Dennis came home for work one Friday evening and Jim said, "I need to talk to you." Dennis knew what Jim was going to say. Jim had lost weight. The nodes in his neck were swollen. He hadn't been feeling good. He'd never complained, but Dennis knew. Jim had told him that morning that he was going to see the doctor. Driving to work Dennis thought, "He has AIDS." For no reason at all.

"We have to talk," Jim said. He sat down at the kitchen table. Dennis sat on the couch.

"Well, the doctor said I have AIDS."

From then on, there wasn't a moment when Dennis was absolutely free of the consciousness that AIDS was in his life.

Dennis felt numb. Jim did most of the talking. He covered their options. They could stay together. He could go back to Texas—he hadn't been living in New York long and he had plenty of friends in Texas. A support system, he called it. He could go back to Texas and not be a burden on Dennis. That's the way Jim put it. Why should he be a burden?

"I don't know what to do," Jim said.

Dennis was numb. They'd been together less than a year. Jim told Dennis he wanted him to take his time, making up his mind.

"I love you," Dennis said. "You love me. We should stay together. I'll take care of you."

Then Dennis went into himself. He thought of suicide. He thought of living out the illness and, when Jim died, killing himself.

The doctor tested Dennis and said he had "perfect blood." He told Jim and Dennis how to have safe sex. But as the months went by, Dennis realized, he didn't want to touch Jim.

"When we first found out," Dennis says, "we kissed and we had safe sex. Then after a while, for some reason, the longer we lived with the disease, I came to a point that I didn't even want to kiss him. I would just get frozen at the thought at night when we were kissing good night."

He would be driving home from work and he would say to himself, Tonight I'm going to make love to Jim. But Jim had lost so much weight. In bed, when Dennis put his arm around Jim, he felt his bones.

There was a drunk-driving commercial on television. The skeleton hand would reach out and grasp the human hand and there would be the sound of the crash in the background. When Jim touched him, Dennis couldn't help it—Jim's hand was like the skeleton hand.

One night, Jim exploded. "I don't know what's going on with us! I don't know if we're roommates, if we're friends, lovers, what!"

"I'm here every day," Dennis said. "I see what's happening to you. It makes me so sad. I'm just so sad. I'm engulfed by it. I'm doing all I can do."

Nothing was resolved. Later that night, lying in bed, Jim said, "I want to tell you something. I'm trying very hard. No one will say, if I die, that I did not go out fighting."

Dennis belongs to a support group for "care partners" at GMHC. Jim says it's shown Dennis that things could be worse, that "he doesn't have such a bad deal after all."

"There are six people in my group," Dennis says. "Half of them have lost most of their friends—because they drifted away when they heard. So these people had to join to get any support. It's the only time they have a chance to talk about it. Most of us are lovers of people with AIDS. Some are in the last stage of the disease.

When I joined the group, one person's lover had died. In the past three months three have died.

"It's wonderful. You go there and you get support. When I talk about what I'm going through and the feelings I'm having, I find out that they're all so normal."

One night in the group, Dennis brought up the fact that he didn't want to touch Jim.

"I'm sure it's just something that everybody's gone through and that you grow out of—a phase."

He told them about the TV commercial.

"Dennis, you're watching too much TV," one man said.

Then they went around the room and everybody in the group told him how important they found touching was—not sex, sex is your own individual thing. But touching, touching and hugging and holding hands. They each said how important it was in their relationship. Even those who had lovers who had died said how important it was at the end, that it became more important.

"Because in some of the hospitals in New York, when they come into your room if you have AIDS," says Dennis, "they wear plastic gloves, they wear plastic masks, they're covered in plastic. Cabrini, where Jim goes, is not that way—they treated him just like any other patient. But the human touch is so important.

"I guess talking about it brought me to the realization of what it was—all in my mind, fear of the disease. Throughout every stage of the disease, that's a major problem. You confuse the disease with the person.

"I drove home and I was mad. I was mad at the other people in the group for not having gone through the same thing. I was mad at myself for having made this up out of nothing.

"Then Friday or Saturday we were sitting watching TV. He was sitting on his corner of the couch and I was at my corner, and I said, 'Come sit by me.' We sat there and cuddled. We hugged and watched TV together. I was relieved. A weight was off my shoulders. I felt good when I went to bed that night—that this was the support I was there to give.

"Jim is slowly becoming an invalid. I used to love to get up on a Saturday morning and we would walk from the Village up to the Metropolitan Museum and then walk through the museum and then walk through the park and then maybe walk down to 42nd Street and get tickets for the theatre that evening. Now the walk is too much for him and so we'll take the subway to the museum. And there are days when he doesn't feel like even walking through the museum because he's too tired.

"I bought him a cane for Valentine's Day. He loved it. He said he was too cheap to go out and buy himself a cane. He needs it to steady himself. One of the symptoms of his illness seems to be that his joints hurt, so his knees hurt. He enjoys walking with it.

"In my mind, I've got a timetable set up—that he's really not going to get seriously ill until after next Christmas. We're going to have a wonderful summer and then he'll probably, as the weather gets cold, start to run down a little bit more. Then maybe in January or February of next year he'll have his first real serious illness. In group everybody said, 'Oh, God should listen to you.'

"As Jim gets sicker and it get closer to the end, Edward will be there to be my support—not my mental support as much as helping me do things for Jim, while he's at the hospital or when he comes home and he's no longer mobile as he is now.

"I've been dealing with this for six months and going to group—so from day one I've been in on it and I've had the time to cry. Not that I'm not sure there isn't a lot more crying left. But I think it's easier for me to be colder about it now, less emotional.

"At least once a week, we've found, there's a little pin, a little thorn, a new added thing. He lost a tooth in bed last night. It just fell out. I'm sure it has nothing to do with

AIDS, but anything that happens you want to blame on AIDS.

"I was wondering aloud in group once if the point would ever come when I would stop bitching about Jim's smoking. I really hate it. And someone whose lover already died said, 'There's a point at which it no longer matters. That's when you've accepted that he's going to die.'

"I see the people in the group. They pretty much keep on an even keel. Even the ones in the group who say, 'I just can't handle it anymore.' The next week they handle more."

Recently a legal adviser from GMHC came to the apartment and drew up a will with Jim. Jim has been looking into cremation.

"When he dies," says Dennis evenly, "I'll have the will. I'll call up the crematorium—if we decide to go with those people. But now is the time to make the decisions." He brightens. "And who knows? Maybe they'll find a cure. And in 20 years when he dies, or 40 years when he dies, it will still be all done."

Dennis says he no longer feels guilty that there are days, or there are moments, when he thinks, "Oh, I just wish Jim would die already." He doesn't really mean he wants Jim to die. He wants the disease to be over with.

Sometimes Jim says, "Not only are we involved in a relationship, we're involved in a gay relationship. I have AIDS. We are dealing with a monumental mountain here that we tidy up every day and go on living with. It's amazing."

Dennis has fantasies of escaping with Jim, but that isn't possible. AIDS will be with both of them forever now.

"I don't think a day goes by that I don't get a pimple and know it's AIDS," Dennis says. "I get a little sore in my mouth because I've bit myself, and it's cancer. But it doesn't last very long. It was a lot worse in the beginning.

It seems that the more you get into it, the easier it gets to accept, the less I think about getting sick. At first I thought all day long, 'Well, I've gotta have it too.'

"I've decided I'm not going to get AIDS. I went through this thing where I was sure I had it. Then I went through this thing that I could never have it. And now—this week—I feel I don't have AIDS and I'm not going to get AIDS from Jim and most probably I will never catch AIDS.

"They say there's up to five-year incubation period before you know whether you have it, so there is a possibility that the virus might be in my body and might be settling in and working away at my blood.

"There is always going to be, from five years since the last time I had sex with Jim intimately, the notion that I have AIDS."

Four years into the epidemic, the emotional tribute AIDS is exacting from the gay community is incalculable. In psychological terms, not just epidemiologically, AIDS has turned out to be like a stone cast into a pond—perhaps diminished, the ripples nevertheless cover the entire surface. No one who comes into contact with AIDS, however healthy in fact, is entirely immune to the havoc it wreaks.

"It gets worse all the time," says Dr. Morin in San Francisco. "You'd think people would adapt to the horror, but it keeps on worsening—there are constantly new levels of horror to adapt to." He says he and his colleagues have identified in their ongoing study a psychiatric "continuum of AIDS-related conditions" analogous to the physical manifestations of the illness. They state that the "psychological impact on gay men is omnipresent and profound."

Not surprisingly, researchers are documenting grief, anger—especially at what is perceived as the inadequate response of government—depression, but most markedly a widespread and unabated anxiety in reaction to AIDS.

Sitting on a time bomb. Living under the gun. Waiting for the other shoe to drop.

"Shell shock" is also a term one often hears. Daily life in the communities AIDS has touched is routinely compared to a combat situation. "You get the feeling you're in Beirut or on the front line of a war," observes Daniel William in New York. Since 1980, 41 of Dr. William's patients have died of AIDS. Thirty-five men in his care have AIDS at present. Two hundred have symptoms of AIDS-Related Complex.

All his homosexual patients, says Dr. William, visit him much more frequently than they did in the past. He emphasizes that few of the "worried well"—whose AIDS- or ARC-like symptoms are often in actuality the classic symptoms of depression—can quite be called hypochondriacal. Under the circumstances, it would be remarkable if the majority didn't feel fragile, vulnerable, endangered.

More gay men are seeking psychotherapy because of AIDS. Dixie Beckham comments that some of her physically well gay clients display levels of anxiety so acute, they "seem almost to be under greater stress than people who have been diagnosed with AIDS."

Commonplace issues of intimacy and coupling have become volatile, pregnant with existential import. Men contemplating a relationship must face a unique uncertainty. They must ask themselves, points out Ms. Beckham, "Does he have AIDS and will I lose him? Do I have AIDS and can I make a commitment to a relationship?" This question, she notes, often must remain "just that—a question."

Each ripple in the media has its repercussions as well. A recent report that the virus might conceivably be transmitted through saliva set off something of a panic. There is lingering confusion as to how one can stay sexually active and not get infected. But even gay men who have adjusted to the probability of already having been infected are buffeted by waves of equivocal messages. Everyone has become his own odds maker.

Now there is a blood test to detect antibodies to the virus thought to cause AIDS but, apart from screening the blood supply, its uses are unclear. The test has also created anxiety and indecision. David Ostrow, head of Chicago's Office of AIDS Activity, says that since it can't in any way diagnose AIDS, "I sometimes think being exposed to the test could be as awful for your health as exposure to the virus."

Psychological burnout among volunteers in organizations like GMHC is chronic. Last February, in the space of two and one-half weeks, six clients attached to Edward's team died. The perpetual cycle of mourning grinds down the strongest sensibility.

Health professionals—gay and heterosexual alike—are themselves hardly exempt from AIDS burnout and anxiety. One psychologist reports that some patients "talk about this lymph node or this swollen gland or that sore throat or that odd-looking spot in their mouth—and at the end of sessions like that I've run into the bathroom to check myself out." General practitioners who are also gay are in a particularly harrowing situation. They're working with patients whom they simply cannot cure and those patients are usually their peers.

There are some rewards. Dr. William says his management of the diseases that commonly accompany AIDS has improved since the nightmare first years of the epidemic to this extent—although he has not been able to add years to patients' lives, "I've added very good months."

6. THE HEART KEEPS BEATING

L ast December, three days after what would have been
their fifth anniversary, Edward visited his lover Robert's grave for the first time.

Robert died at New York Hospital on December 22,
1983, from *pneumocystis* pneumonia, Kaposi's sarcoma, and
host of other illnesses.

Robert's final hospital stay lasted four months. Edward
visited him every afternoon. If Robert's family visited,
they came in the evening. Robert was not "out" to his
family. He had not told them he was gay. Edward was
known as "Robert's friend."

The cemetery is in a pastoral setting about an hour
from New York City. Edward's friend Bob drove him
there. It was a beautiful day, clear, sunny. At the cemetery office, the secretary, not realizing that the plat was
upside down, had a lot of trouble locating Robert's grave.
Then she made a real production out of telling Edward
how to reach it—until it occurred to her to take him to
the window. She pointed out the grave. It was about 100
feet away. Bob waited in the car.

The cemetery is well maintained. There are graveled

paths and manicured lawns. The shrubs were bare but there were no leaves on the ground.

Robert's stone is very simple—red marble, smooth on its face, with Robert's name and dates chiseled out in Roman letters. There was a moment of sadness because of the dates—so few years between them. But Edward knew immediately, Robert was not there.

Edward was relieved. He'd had visions of turning into the kind of person who religiously tends a grave. He stood there looking down at the stone.

I wondered probably what everyone who has ever lost a mate wonders—does anybody really know how much I've lost? I'm very self sufficient. Maybe I don't encourage people to be sympathetic. But would anybody ever be able to acknowledge the depth of my loss? Standing there, looking down at the tombstone, it became so real to me, how intense the loss is. The truth may be that nobody else can acknowledge a loss like that. That may be the truth.

Every day when Edward had visited the hospital, he'd taken Robert a red carnation. It was the flower he'd always given Robert. After standing by the grave a while, Edward lay a red carnation at the base of the stone and left.

Several weeks after he visited Robert's grave, Edward called Robert's mother, as he sometimes does. "By the way," he said, "I went to the cemetery."

"I know," she said.

"But how did you know?"

"I saw the carnation."

It had never crossed his mind that she might have known—he was, of course, the one who brought Robert a carnation every day. Now, Edward saw, she'd known that and perhaps more, but could never have said what she knew.

It began with what they thought was a bruise. It was a Kaposi's sarcoma lesion.

When it came to really serious, big things, he wasn't a great communicator. I would have to draw him out. He didn't deny he had AIDS but he denied the fact that it was fatal. Initially he was optimistic. Then, after several trips in and out of the hospital and having to leave work and severe weight loss and the beginning of a series of devastating parasitic infections—he just stopped communicating on an emotional level.

When Robert was diagnosed with AIDS, in the fall of 1982, not much was known about the disease. This encouraged Robert in his optimism. "Don't worry about it," he would tell Edward. "We're going to beat it."

Robert was treated for Kaposi's sarcoma at New York Hospital and the cancer went into remission. He went back to work. Robert was a social worker in a nonprofit agency. A lot of people depended on him.

I saw him go through something I'm seeing Jim go through now—that time when he had to remove himself from the rest of the world. He had a real hard time. He took his work seriously. When he could no longer do it, that bothered him.

We did a lot of lying to each other—I would agree that all he needed was some time off.

Over the next year, Robert had *pneumocystis* pneumonia a number of times. He developed toxoplasmosis, an opportunistic infection that causes brain abscesses. He had constant diarrhea "which he found so humiliating. He never got over it." He had skin rashes. He suffered nerve damage from a herpetic lesion at the base of his spine. His feet were swollen from an edemalike condition—both of these made walking increasingly difficult.

He'd had terrible problems walking and I got him a cane. I thought it would cheer him up. It was very elaborate, with a dog's head handle. It was a fancy walking stick, as opposed to a sickroom cane. He didn't seem to care one way or the other.

One day we met for lunch. He came into the city—he'd been staying with his parents—and he was at the restaurant when I got there. When we finished and stood up—I hadn't seen him for three days or so—the deterioration was so pronounced. It took us almost half an hour to walk three quarters of a block.

On Labor Day weekend, Edward took Robert to the hospital in an ambulance.

He was in intensive care and hooked up to a respirator. I didn't have clearance to visit him in intensive care because I wasn't acknowledged as anything but a friend.

A wonderful nurse there dressed me up like a doctor—she put a stethoscope around my neck, handed me a clipboard, and we bullied our way into intensive care. The reason I did it is because things were looking very bad and I thought I had to see him. So I went in.

He was in this very small room. He was surrounded with tubes and machines. He opened his eyes and the nurse said, 'He doesn't know you're here.'

But I knew him so well. He looked surprised to see me. He couldn't talk because he had this mask over his mouth. I said, 'I know you can't talk, but if you understand what I'm saying, wiggle your eyebrows.'

And he started wiggling his eyebrows. We had this little conversation, just the two of us, which he never remembered—but at the time it was wonderful.

When Robert got out of intensive care, Edward visited him every day from one to four in the afternoon, so they could be alone together. The doctor had told Robert's family he had AIDS. Just as Robert was able to acknowledge that he had AIDS but not that it was fatal, his family knew Robert was dying of AIDS but never were able to acknowledge that he was gay. At one time, Robert had been married and his mother was sure he was going to marry again.

It's hard to say which kind of denial created more pain for Edward, but as it gradually became apparent that Robert would never leave the hospital, Edward needed to say good-bye.

I wanted to talk to him about how much he had meant to me, about how much I would miss him. And I wanted to hear that from him. And yet, talking about someone's death is a place you have to be invited into. He couldn't let anybody in there.

He wanted to get out of the hospital so bad. I think I would have just picked him up, gone down in the elevator, got him into a cab, and brought him home. He wanted out so badly. But you listen to doctors giving advice and the residents and you're so concerned with getting him well that as long as there's a possibility you just—

And then, in the middle of all this, this incredible black comedy-like event took place. He told me he didn't like the physical therapist who was assigned to come in and try to help him walk. He said she treated him like a child. He said he wouldn't mind getting up and walking around for a while. So I said, 'Why don't I help you get out of the bed and let's just have you walk from the bed to the chair and sit in the chair for a while?' He said he'd try it—he hadn't been out of bed in weeks.

I was never fully aware of the expression 'dead weight' before— here I am with this man who at that point weighed about 100 pounds but it seemed like 1,000. I'm holding him up because his feet aren't supporting him and I have this IV rack in one hand and all I can think is that it's like something out of an insane English movie—we're just going to go sprawling onto the floor.

So I started to laugh and he started to laugh. It must have been painful but it gave him a laugh. It was one of the last genuine moments of intimacy we had together.

As AIDS stepped up its attack on his brain, Robert's behavior became arbitrary and capricious. Before Edward left for the hospital, he would call Robert on the phone.

"I'm on my way over. What can I get for you?"

"I want a potato knish and a salami."

"Okay, you want a potato knish and some salami."

"No, not some salami—I want a salami."

Edward would arrive with the food.

"I can't eat."

It was almost as if Robert needed to see if he could still

summon things up, manifest some power in the midst of his growing powerlessness.

Edward phoned Robert every night to say good night. In the last few months, however, Robert refused to answer the phone. At 10 o'clock Edward would have to call the nurses' station and ask a nurse to go into Robert's room. Then, when Edward rang Robert's number again, she would pick up the receiver and hand it to Robert. Maybe this was Robert's way of exercising some final small measure of control.

About a month before Robert died, he became paranoid.

"Why'd you let them change my room? Why'd you let them put me in a smaller room?"

"Robert, you're in the same room."

"No I'm not."

He would accuse the nurses of putting something in his food.

At times, Robert was borderline psychotic. But he was so weak, he couldn't be violent.

I don't want to see the things I've seen.

The last few weeks Robert was in the hospital, Edward desperately wanted him to die. Robert was no longer the person Edward had known. He could not walk. He weighed 60 pounds. He was blind. He had lost his hearing. He was in an almost constant state of epileptic seizure. He could not speak. He would not die.

Robert's doctor, a young resident, simply stopped coming to see him. Robert's mother had agreed to let him die. There was no plug to pull or Edward would have pulled it. Robert's body would not die. Edward stood by helplessly. Moving around Robert's room, the nurses refused to say anything negative about his condition. "Who knows what he can hear?" one of them told Edward outside in the hall. "We don't think he can hear anything but who knows?"

The day before Robert finally did die, Edward watched while the nurse changed his gown. Beneath the withered skin, under the rib cage, Edward could see Robert's heart, its outline. He could see it beating.

When Robert died, Edward's years with him got canceled out in one stroke. He didn't go to Robert's funeral. He was invited to the funeral but Edward says he couldn't share Robert any longer. He could no longer pretend for Robert's sake in front of Robert's family that they were not lovers.*

AIDS isn't like cancer, Edward says. Cancer is frightening but respectable, he says. His gay friends, when Robert died, wanted desperately for Edward to bounce back. They didn't encourage him to talk to them about Robert's death. They didn't want to deal with the fact that Robert had died of AIDS. "AIDS was a dark, terrifying pit they didn't want to look into," says Edward.

It was interesting—Edward began to notice that no one would touch him, with the exception of one woman he knew who made a point of reaching out and grabbing him and hugging him.

Edward went into a state of business as usual. He prided himself on his self-control and strength. What he really wanted was to just let go and have someone catch him.

Robert died at Christmastime. People later told Edward that he behaved during the holidays as if he were doing perfectly well. Maybe he did. Everybody, he thought, was suddenly very busy.

About two weeks after Robert died, Edward's friend Bob called and said, "I want to see you, let's get together."

They met for lunch and Edward suddenly found himself feeling very edgy. Bob hadn't yet found the time to sit down with him and talk about Robert's death. He'd always seemed to have too many things to do. Edward was edgy.

---

*Even now Edward feels he must keep Robert's secret. Robert is not the real name of Edward Dunn's dead lover.

They ordered.

"You're really pissed off at me," Bob said. "Aren't you?"

Edward looked at him. "Yeah, I really am." He realized it when Bob said it.

"Why?"

Edward was incredulous. "Because you just disappeared for two weeks."

Bob weighed that. "Edward, what do you want to say to me?"

And Edward screamed—*"Where were you?"*

He held onto the edge of the table and let it out. Bob didn't seem surprised. People turned to look at them. Edward began to shake.

"I got it," Bob said.

Edward began to cry.

The truth was, Robert was all Edward wanted to talk about. He wanted to sit in a room without sleep and babble incoherently every detail he had ever known about Robert. He wanted to talk about Robert and nothing else.

Edward sought out a bereavement counselor through GMHC. Edward's counselor encouraged him to remember Robert before his illness and disintegration. He encouraged Edward to pay attention to his dreams, because Edward's unconscious was helping him to mourn. He encouraged Edward to bring mementos of Robert into their sessions. He encouraged Edward to talk to Robert and say what he hadn't been able to say when Robert was alive. He encouraged Edward to say good-bye.

Edward volunteered to work at GMHC. His bereavement counselor says that although Edward wasn't able to save Robert, he will be able, through helping others, at least to retrace his steps.

A few months after Robert died, Edward went through a period—it lasted about a week—of acute anxiety about having AIDS. It was a reaction he hadn't allowed himself all the time Robert was ill. When Robert was alive, Edward was always very careful not to show any personal concern about AIDS. He didn't want Robert to have to deal with any feelings of guilt he might have about the possibility that Edward might be infected as well. "We never speculated on which one of us might have brought AIDS into the relationship. Certainly, neither of us had ever been particularly promiscuous."

"I was just unlucky," Robert once said.

7. IN THE PLANE OF ACCEPTANCE

When Jim Sharp was diagnosed with *pneumocystis* pneumonia in December 1984, he refused to go into the hospital.

It came upon him in Atlantic City. They were on the boardwalk when Jim turned to Dennis and said, "I've got to go home now. I can't stand up." He knew it was pneumonia.

The next day Jim got up, took a shower, and put on a suit, intending to drop by the doctor's office on his way to work.

Jim had all the symptoms that accompany *pneumocystis carinii* pneumonia—shortness of breath, congestion, coughing, tightness in the chest, fever. Routinely, patients with these symptoms are hospitalized and undergo a nonsurgical procedure called a bronchoscopy to extract a tissue sample from the lung. At first, his doctor thought he was joking, but Jim insisted on forgoing the test and being treated as an outpatient.

Since Jim's condition wasn't critical, his doctor acquiesced and prescribed one of the standard medications for *pneumocystis* pneumonia. If Jim's symptoms went away, he reasoned, that would constitute diagnosis and treatment of the disease in one stroke. If Jim felt worse, he could go into the hospital later. His doctor had already seen how Jim reacted to hospitalization—not well. "Jim always does better outside the hospital," his doctor notes.*

The drug "hit me like a sledgehammer," Jim says. "I felt like someone had run over me, as if I'd been beaten to a pulp." He'd never felt so sick in his life. Then, to top it off, he woke up one morning and his face was covered with herpes zoster blisters. The blisters were extremely painful. And yet Jim dragged himself into work, if only for two or three hours a day. "Consequently," Jim says, "I worked myself out of work."

It took Jim a month to begin to recover, but he was able to keep the true nature of his illness a secret. Some days he was so tired it took all his energy to say a single sentence. He was putting things off—taking a folder out of a desk drawer to make a notation, for instance—because he was so exhausted. Another disturbing phenomenon manifested itself. Jim was forgetting things. "You've said that sixteen times before," Dennis would tell him.

Finally, after Christmas, his doctor told Jim he had a choice. He could either work at full capacity and die, or cut back and live.

Edward remembers, Jim told him beforehand, coolly and rationally, that he was going to meet with his boss to tell him he had AIDS. He was going to tell him he had

---

*Since Jim's doctor didn't take a biopsy and there was no physical evidence per se that Jim had *pneumocystis* pneumonia, at this juncture Jim still hadn't been officially diagnosed with AIDS. Partly as a result of instances like this, the extent of AIDS was chronically underreported in the early years of the epidemic. Aside from the usual obstacles that confront statisticians, the Centers for Disease Control was hampered by doctors who didn't report documented cases even after death and its retention of a narrow 1981 definition of the disease led to numbers that didn't jibe with the profile of AIDS that was emerging. Later in 1985, the C.D.C. expanded its definition to include lymphoma and a few other AIDS-associated conditions that physicians widely considered to be markers of severe acquired immune deficiency—if the patient also tested positive for the HIV antibody.

AIDS and try to negotiate a way for him to ease off. Jim
was very cool about it. Then suddenly, the morning of
the meeting, Jim was on the phone, in a complete panic.

"I don't know what I'm going to do. I have to go in
and see the boss. I have to tell him I'm gay, I have to tell
him I have AIDS." Jim was almost babbling. "I don't
know what I'm going to say."

Gradually, Edward calmed him down. They arranged
to meet at a coffee shop near Jim's office before his
appointment that afternoon.

When Edward arrived, Jim was nervously waiting in a
booth. The restaurant was virtually empty.

"Did you order anything?"

"No." Jim was smoking up a storm.

The waiter came. Edward ordered coffee. "What are
you going to have?" Edward asked Jim.

"Coffee, I guess."

"You have to put something in your stomach. How
about—rice pudding?"

"I'm not hungry."

"Have some rice pudding."

"Why?"

"Because mother says so."

Jim laughed. He visibly relaxed.

They went over his options. At the end of half an hour,
they'd come up with a scheme for Jim to present to his
boss—Jim could at least finish up his current projects
working out of his apartment.

"So I'll go in and tell him I'm sorry that this has—"

"Don't tell him you're sorry, Jim. It isn't your fault you
have AIDS. Okay?"

When it was time to go, Edward paid the check and
walked Jim as far as the lobby of his office building. With
a wave of his hand, Jim disappeared into the elevator.

That evening he called Edward. "He is truly a wonderful man," Jim said. "It was very emotional. He said he

thought I was gay. He said he was afraid it was AIDS. He said he's been praying all along it wasn't."

Jim was elated. How many bosses would sit down with you and try to work out a way to keep you on if you walked in and told them you had AIDS?

Edward was tremendously relieved. He congratulated Jim. But then, when they'd hung up, Edward thought of Robert—how hard Robert took it when he had to quit his job, how Robert never lost hope, how Robert never stopped believing that someday he would go back to work.

Jim and Edward haven't talked about Robert yet. They talk about movies, books, the theatre—ordinary things, because for now they have what passes for an ordinary relationship, and the ordinariness of it is what they've accomplished together so far.

Edward says, "We'll be talking on the phone and Jim will say, 'I love you and I'm glad you're in my life.' That's a wonderful acknowledgment. It's usually toward the end of the conversation and it's not like some flip sign-off. He says a lot of things offhandedly but he says this in a way so as to be sure I get it."

Jim says, "Edward calls me every day and jokes with me. He tells me not to scrub floors, let Dennis do it, after all what are lovers for? He tells me not to kick any old ladies on the street or drown any kittens. He's really saying, Rest, try not to get too upset. I know he cares about me. I've never been so grateful to have somebody in my life."

They have discussed God, mortality, and eternity, but not the prospect of Jim's death—not yet, not seriously.

Edward feels that soon he will have to begin reminding himself that Jim's body is not Jim.

Jim feels he is absolutely going to beat this disease.

Sometimes they joke about death. Jim will even joke about Dennis's next lover. The jokes are sometimes mordant, sometimes campy, sometimes tasteless. They're a safety valve. They mask the fear and corrosive rage that are now as firmly rooted in Jim as is the virus itself. They're a leveler. They're a way of masking the fundamental injustice that lies at the core of Jim's and Edward's relationship—that it just as easily could have been Edward and not Jim.

But it is Jim. And the prospect of Jim's death is like a vast rampart they are approaching. It circumscribes their relationship as surely as does Jim's fierce will to survive. The question isn't whether this prospect can be demolished or even surmounted, but whether Edward can help Jim stay on this side of it.

February 15. Pockmarked snow lies unmelted in the gutters but the sun is out today. From his window, Jim watches the old women and winos skirt the shadows on the sidewalk. They adhere fastidiously to the fringe of sunlight along the curb. He is like them, treading a fine line.

There is a steady rasp from the radiator under the window. Trucks pass by, the windowpanes groan. Down the street, near Our Lady of Pompeii, children let out of school shriek and chirp.

Jim often thinks—if this apartment were on the back of the building, maybe facing a brick wall, he'd go berserk.

Today is officially his last day. For the first time since he went to work at twelve in a little country store in Texas, he will be out of work.

The other day the woman from GMHC came by and helped him with the applications for disability insurance.

A little while ago, the intercom buzzed. It was Frank, the office messenger. "Yo-bro!" Frank said, and stepped in. He turned off his tape machine and removed his headphones and probably for the last time handed Jim the interoffice mail.

They'd told Jim that Frank was bringing down his paycheck but it was not in the envelope. Jim needs that check. Yesterday he was lassoing markets like a world champion calf roper. Tomorrow he will be pulling down zero.

There are two phones in this apartment. Often during the past few weeks Jim has found himself talking on both of them at the same time. Jim loves his work.

Jim called Edward and told him about the check, then he unplugged both of the phones.

He's only 34 and he can feel the fires going out in his body. The medicine cabinet, which for a year contained no pill bottles, is now full of them. But it's interesting—he still doesn't look like a person with AIDS is supposed to look, or at least the way people think you look.

Jim's "numbers" are pretty good. Jim's doctor says he can show you people walking on the edge of the cliff, people who have no immunity to anything and who nevertheless feel great, people who still go to the gym and work out, people who run around the park. Turn the coin over, there is Jim Sharp. Some days, he can't get out of bed.

Jim isn't afraid of death but he is afraid of what dying might entail. What he's most afraid of is seeing Dennis cry, seeing Edward sad. Sometimes he thinks it's very selfish on his part. He doesn't want to hurt the people who love him. Each night when he goes to bed he thanks God for his sobriety and asks for sobriety for the remainder of this day and all his tomorrows. He asks God to please not let him live in hysteria but in the plane of acceptance.

He's been lucky. His lover didn't leave him. He's stopped asking Dennis, Are you sure? They haven't been evicted from their apartment. Jim lost some friends—one woman told him that if he felt good about himself he wouldn't be sick. He made some friends.

He wants to be back in the office in the middle of it all but he thinks now he will probably never go back again.

He knows now, he will have to live with this.

1986

And when he had spent all, there arose a mighty famine in that land; and he began to be in want.
—The Gospel of St. Luke

GREELEY, COLORADO

This is a story about a mother's love for a son who was lost, then found, then lost again forever. It begins on a spring morning in 1974. The father is driving down a country road on his way to work when he sees his son's clothes scattered all over the road. He even runs over some of them before he's able to stop the car.

There's a red backpack at the side of the road that belongs to his son. So do the jeans, T-shirts, socks, and underwear lying on the road and in the ditch. The father picks up his son's clothes and stuffs them into the backpack.

At home, the mother tries not to worry too much. This isn't the first time her son has got drunk and disappeared. Maybe he got in a fight. Maybe the cops will call and tell her to come pick him up. But where was he taking his clothes?

The son has two friends in the world, two older boys who rent a house on the other side of town. Maybe they're brothers, maybe not—no one knows for sure. So the next day, the mother goes out there. The house is empty.

She asks the neighbor lady, "Don't they still live there?"

"They left, I don't know when," the neighbor lady says.

"I think, though, they were evicted, on account of the noise and the drugs." The two women shake their heads in dismay.

Now the mother is really scared. Her son is only 17. He's a little, skinny boy. These boys her son hangs out with are older than him, almost men. She knows her son drinks with these men. He smokes grass with them. Now what if they did something to her son?

The worried parents call the cops but the cops say they can't do anything—you have to wait so many days before they'll fill out a missing persons report. The parents quiz their other children. They call all their sisters and brothers here and in other states. They rack their brains for clues.

Months pass and still no word from their son. The cops just shrug their shoulders and say, Kids, what can you do? The parents still expect that the phone will ring any day now and it will be their son joking around.

Years pass and the parents fear the worst. There's really no reason not to.

1. TO BE FREE

When Nellie got married the first time, her father said, "You made your bed, you lie in it."

This was in 1955. Nellie was 15 years old. Her new husband was 22. All she knew was, she wanted a home. Nellie was one of twelve children. After her mother died, when Nellie was 8, she and her younger brothers and sisters were raised like orphans. They lived in foster homes here, there, and everywhere—like stray dogs. All Nellie ever wanted was to be able to say, I can stay here tonight and I can stay here tomorrow night and I can stay here next week.

At 15, she thought, I'm so smart, I'm going to get married. She didn't have any schooling. She spoke broken English and broken Spanish. Chicanos and Anglos alike would ask her, Where are you from? From here, she'd say, embarrassed. This is long, long before she went to the community college and took English lessons.

By the time she was 21, Nellie had 5 kids. She grew up with her kids. She did everything with them. They had picnics. They went to the movies. They played games. They played hide-and-go-seek, jacks, hopscotch. They wrassled. They played football. If she was pregnant or

not pregnant, she played with her kids. They had snow-
ball fights. She did somersaults on the bed with them,
imagine—a married woman. But she was just a kid herself. For a long time it was just Nellie and her kids. She
had nothing else.

There was Mary, the oldest, then Mike, then Larry,
Dolores, and Rudy.

Nellie's husband was there but he wasn't there. He
worked in the daytime during the week and over the
weekend he was drunk or he was gone. He would get
paid on Friday and he would leave, then he'd come back
Monday morning. When they were first married, he tried
to get Nellie to drink with him but she didn't care for it.

"You know what you are, old woman? You're a drag.
Come on, you're holding me back here."

They were poor. It was a hard life. It was a bad marriage, but whenever Nellie thought of leaving her husband, she thought, Where am I going to go with all these
kids? What am I going to do? I can't work. This was long
before she started to get out in the world.

So Nellie raised these five kids by herself. She made
lots of mistakes she was sorry for later. But no one ever
raised Nellie, so how was she to know how you raise five
kids? She had a terrible temper and sometimes she hit
them. When she was at the end of her rope, she probably
hit them more than she should have.

When the kids got to be teenagers, that's when the
problems began. There was a fight in the house every
day. Nellie was strict. She was picky. Everything had to be
just the way she said or else. Her kids wondered, What
happened? Mom wasn't any fun anymore. Other kids
might run in packs but Nellie wouldn't let hers go. She
would not let them go. When her kids wanted to go out
and do all the things teenagers do, Nellie said no. When
they complained, Everybody else gets to, she would reply,
I didn't. Nellie was bitter. It was like, I never got to, why
should you?

Their father wasn't any help. Even when he was home, he didn't have any time for his kids. Nellie would say, "You have to talk to them, you have to talk to your kids. If you don't talk to them, what kind of a life are they going to have? What are we going to tell our grandkids, when they get older and they ask what happened and we can't tell them nothing good?"

And yet, her husband favored Mike. Mike was the oldest boy. Mike could do no wrong. If Mike did something wrong, the other kids got blamed for it. So Mike always had to have his own way. He grew up always having to be right even if he wasn't.

When Mike was little, he was very bright, he could make you laugh. Then gradually, as he grew older, she noticed, her son was a loner. He wrote poems. He drew pictures. He read books. He kept to himself. He had this album of birds—pictures of birds he'd cut out of magazines and such, pictures of birds he drew himself. No one was allowed to touch it. No one could touch Mike's stuff but him. He would never share. He was tight, he was stingy. He hoarded every little bit of money he could get his hands on. Everything of his was his and everything had to be just so.

His bird book and all the poems of his she kept? They got wrecked when the basement flooded that time.

She knew he was gay. Maybe she should have said something, but she thought he would grow out of it. He never would work in the yard with his brothers. He would do anything—cook or wash dishes, do any kind of housework, not to mow the lawn. She noticed, he liked more of the female sort of thing. He would take his money and buy stationery with perfume on it. He was always with girls.

So the other kids teased him. She knew because his sisters and brothers came home and told her. And she would be cleaning the house and she'd find notes he had saved in his drawer or even left out on the top of the dresser.

STAY AWAY FROM US YOU SISSIE
IF YOU KNOW WHAT'S GOOD FOR YOU

Mike must have left these notes out in the open like that because he wanted her to find them, but she never brought it up.

Mike had a lot of problems at school. By this time she was working at the school, so she saw. He got picked on a lot. The other kids picked on him, the teachers picked on him. She told them, I work here eight hours a day and I see. In her bones, she knew things weren't right with her son. But when the school psychologist tried to talk to her about the gay part, she refused. She just couldn't.

Years later Nellie would lie awake at night and wonder, What if I did different? What if I did different? The mother always gets the blame. But she did wonder.

Years later her son threw it up to her—that it was her fault, that she didn't accept him for what he was. Mike knew how to reach in, how to drill in, how to prick that aching spot where Nellie's doubt lay. She would defend herself. She would retort, You don't accept you yourself. But she wondered and it made her cry.

Whatever. By the time he was 16, Mike was running around a lot and she couldn't do anything with him. All the kids did that. That was their thing. They would get in a car and go off and get drunk, raise heck. This was when they were still living in Kersey, outside of Greeley. Mike would get drunk at the park in Greeley and his father would have to go in and pick him up. It was ten miles away.

"What are you doing to yourself, getting drunk all the time like this?"

"Oh, Mom, Dad drinks, too, you know."

Then he met those two guys and he started hanging out with them and taking drugs, L.S.D. and pot.

"You'd better be careful with the drugs and all that."

"Oh, Mom," Mike said, "everybody does that."

When Mike was 17, he dropped out of school. She asked him what he was going to do if he didn't go to school.

"You know, Mom, I'd just like to live on the streets."

"How come you want to do that?"

"You always have me tied here at home and I want to be free. I don't want no one to boss me around, to tell me ever again what to do. I'm tired of you telling me what to do. I want to go live and not work for anybody and live on the street. And when I'm free, if I want to work I will and if I don't want to I won't."

She thought this was just hippie talk. "I think you should get a job," she said. "Settle down, make something of your life."

"Oh, Mom, that's what you think. But that's not what I want."

Whatever. Then he decided to get his diploma. Oh, he was smart. He went to the community college and got his equivalency diploma. Just like that. It gave her some hope.

But no, her son was adrift. They got him a job at the slaughterhouse but he only went one day.

"What do you think, I'm crazy?"

His father got him a job at Kodak but he never showed up. He was running around with those other boys. He was high all the time. He was stealing things to buy his drugs and his marijuana. She knew that. Things came up missing.

Then he was gone and they didn't know what had happened to him and it was too late.

After five years, in 1979, the phone rings and it's her son.

"But where are you?"

Each time Mike calls, his father sends money through the mail to a different post office. Mike keeps moving from state to state. This goes on for months and months, then, when there isn't any more money to send Mike, he comes home.

He is a bitter person. Who knows what her son has seen?

"But how did you live?"

"On the streets, but I don't wanna talk about it, okay?"

"But why did you run away?" his mother asks him.

"Oh, Mom, you never understand. To be free."

"And now do you feel free living like this, like you're telling me, on the street, where you do?"

"You know, Mom, I'm gay," he tells Nellie, as if that's the reason.

"I knew you were gay, a long time," his mother says, "since you were a young boy. I love you just the same."

This makes him furious. "Don't bullshit me. I know you hate me because I'm gay. I hate the way I am, too. But you know, Mom, it's your fault. You brought me into this world. You raised me this way. You made my life hell. Why didn't you get rid of me when I was born?"

Sometimes her son sits staring. Sometimes he laughs when there's nothing to laugh at. He won't work. He only wants to take drugs. Nellie and his father discuss it—how can they have him? It's worse than before. Finally, Mike's father says, That's it, he goes.

No one wants her son. His sisters and brothers don't want him. His father doesn't want him. What can Nellie do? She asks Mike where he wants to go and buys him a ticket with her own money.

At the bus depot, Mike says to her, "All this is your fault. It's your fault my father won't give me any more money."

"Whatever you want to think," Nellie tells him. "We

don't have it anymore. We sent you all the money we had. It can't be that way anymore."

"You're no longer my family," he says. "You're no longer my mother."

"We're still your family."

"No, because I disown you. You never accepted me the way I was."

What can she say?

Two, three years later, Mike calls.

"You know where I am, you old bitch? I'm on the street again." He is drunk or on drugs or both. "And you know why I'm on the street again, you bitch? That's what you wanted for me, not to be anything, to live this life." He carries on like that.

This becomes a habit. When Mike calls, he always calls collect and curses her but Nellie never hangs up. "Please don't talk to me this way anymore," she says. "Give me your number and I'll call you." Maybe he doesn't have a phone. Whatever. He won't. Or if he does, they've never heard of him there.

One night he calls and he's happy. He says he is living with rich people. He says he's going to send his mother glassware and some expensive jewelry. She doesn't believe any of this. He's never even sent a Christmas card.

Sometimes he gets drunk and calls the whole family, his aunts and uncles, cousins. The phone company contacts his aunt in California about a stolen credit card.

One night he calls his mother and says, "I need that $6,000."

"What $6,000?" she asks.

"I sent you $6,000."

"From where? Where did you get $6,000?"

"That's what you bought your house with, you fucking bitch!"

She tries to stay calm. "You're mistaken. We haven't got anything. We haven't even heard from you."

He likes to keep hammering at her until she's in tears. Then he says, "I gotcha, Mom, I gotcha!" and hangs up.

"Why are you doing this to me?" she cries. "What did I do to you?"

"You never loved me. I used to give you presents, remember? And you threw them in the trash. You didn't even unwrap them, Mom, and you threw them in the trash."

"I never, I never did that."

"Just like you threw me in the trash, Mom. Here I am in the trash."

When Mike's sisters and brothers were all grown up, Nellie looked around and said, There isn't anything here for me. She divorced their father.

"You're just a whore," Mike said on the phone. "No wonder my father divorced you."

"You know your father used to drink, you know he ran around. You know me. You know how I was. I wasn't a whore. You're sick, you know. You need to see someone about your sickness."

"Well, you made me this way, Mom, huh?"

Nellie met Mr. Rocha and married him.

"If you think I'm gonna accept any bastard for my father," Mike screamed through the phone, "think again, Mom, you think again!"

"You have a father," Nellie told him. "You don't need a father. I didn't marry somebody else to be your father. Look, if this is what you're calling for, don't call me anymore. You're a complete stranger."

"You gonna cry now, Ma? Oh-oh, there she goes. She's gonna cry. Now she's crying. Boo-hoo. Okay, Ma. Bye, Ma. Bye-bye."

In March 1986, Mike called his mother. "You know what, Mom?" He was calling from San Francisco. "They're gonna check me for AIDS now."

"You're kidding. Why do you kid me like this?"

"No, I'm serious." But he was laughing.

"Are you sick?"

"I was sick. I was real weak but I'm not sick no more."

"Well, why are they checking you for the AIDS then?"

"I don't know."

"Why are you laughing? Is this another one of your pranks, that you're calling and making me worry?"

"Oh, Mom, you know I like to rile you." He is still laughing. "Well, Mom, I'll let you know," Mike says and hangs up.

2. VERY GOOD
AND BEAUTIFUL DAY

O n April 24, 1986, Michael Maes appeared at San
Francisco General Hospital. He stank so, it was hard
to sit in the same room with him.

Mike had been referred to Ward 86, part of the hospital's AIDS service, from a public health clinic in the heart
of the Castro, San Francisco's "gay ghetto." Because of its
large gay population, San Francisco had been hit hard by
AIDS early on. By the spring of 1986, over 2,500 cases
had been diagnosed in the metropolitan area. One 1984
study had estimated that 65 percent of the gay males in
the city had been infected by the HIV virus.

Doctors and administrators at San Francisco General
were quick to realize that people with AIDS, because of
their unique social and medical problems, required specialized care in an environment where the staff was unusually knowledgeable and sympathetic, so they moved to
centralize and coordinate services. The result was Ward
5A and its outpatient arm, Ward 86. When the so-called
AIDS ward was established, early in 1983, critics said it
would be seen as a leper colony—patients, their families
and friends would shun treatment there. But these fears

proved to be unfounded. Soon over half the people with AIDS in the city were being served by it.

Mike was seen first at the outpatient clinic by Lauren Poole, a nurse-practitioner, and Kevin Burke, a social worker. Mike told them he'd been living in a hotel on Sixth Street, in a seedy part of the Mission district, but the hotel had burned down and now he was sleeping on the street. He avoided the city shelters, he said, because he was afraid of getting beaten and robbed. He was dirty but he wasn't filthy. His clothes stank. Mr. Burke went out to find some new shoes and socks for Mike.

Mike made an indelible impression on Nurse Poole. Sitting before her was a small, sweet, unassuming man with bright black eyes, homeless and alone, who told her his sad story without embellishment.

Mike was 29 years old, Mexican-American, and gay. He was born in Greeley, Colorado. His father and mother, now divorced, still lived in Greeley. He had two brothers and two sisters as well. Mike said he'd never been on good terms with his mother and ran away from home at 17 because she had a hard time dealing with his gayness. He hadn't, he said, seen any of his family for 12 years.

Mike didn't disclose a visit home in 1979, the year he lived with his aunt in California, or many other details of his wanderings since he'd left home. In a subsequent psychiatric interview, however, he revealed that he had a history of manic-depressive illness that began, he said, before he ran away and had resulted over the years in a number of confused periods. He reported four suicide attempts. The first time, Mike tried to overdose on aspirin. The last time, two years before, he tried to kill himself by jumping off a bridge. In the past he'd been treated with lithium and Desyrel but, he said, he'd often quit his medication in order to drink. He'd always recognized the onset of illness and was able to get help. Although he said he hadn't been taking any psychotropic medication for eight months, Mike seemed to the psychiatrist who inter-

viewed him to be balanced, alert, and aware. Throughout
his hospital stay, Mike's behavior was deemed "appropri-
ate" and he was termed a cooperative patient.

Mike had been in San Francisco for two and a half
years. Before that, he said, he lived in New Orleans,
Minneapolis, Iowa, Nevada, and in other parts of California. He'd worked in an office in New Orleans, he said, but
otherwise had never held down a full-time job. He said
he'd been a part-time day laborer in San Francisco.

In March, out of curiosity, Mike said, he took the test
for the AIDS antibody. He tested positive. At the time, he
felt okay, but lately he'd been feeling tired. For the past
three weeks, he'd been waking up in the middle of the
night soaked with sweat. He estimated that he'd lost 20
pounds in the past month. Sometimes he had a pounding
headache. He had a dry cough. There was something
else—he was shy about mentioning it to a woman.

On examination, Nurse Poole took a culture and treated
Mike for rectal herpes. He was very grateful for the
Acyclovir cream she gave him as he said his ass had hurt
for two months. Partly because of the pain, partly because
of the fatigue, it had taken him, he said, two hours to
walk from the Tenderloin to the hospital—a distance of
about two miles.

Mike readily volunteered the fact that he was alcoholic and customarily drank up to three fifths of wine a
day. "I've been drunk every day for the past ten years,"
he said with a shrug. "But you know, I never had the
d.t.'s or anything." He'd been through four different
alcohol rehabilitation programs and most recently was in
contact with the Ozanam program of the St. Vincent de
Paul Society, on Howard Street, a detoxification center.
He hadn't gone through the program there but, he said,
he hadn't had a drink since March.

There were, in fact, lots of indications that Mike was
working hard to bring his often chaotic life into focus
again. In March, he'd also registered for food stamps. He

carried check-cashing cards, a social security card, and a photo identification card issued by the Department of Motor Vehicles.

Mike said he'd gone to a lot of bars on Polk Street and met a lot of men but he was tired of that now and ready to make a change. He'd been in a monogamous relationship for three years, he said, but had been sexually promiscuous—that was the word he used—for the past six months.

Mike struck Nurse Poole as being honest and intelligent. Moreover, he had a sense of humor about himself and his circumstances. "Huggable," she thought, sitting there listening to him. She could tell that although Mike appeared passive and weak, he was good at getting people to take care of him. Wasn't Kevin out right now trying to hustle up a tent and a sleeping bag? Nurse Poole wondered—she'd had many opportunities to test her judgment about these things, and she wondered if in Mike's case getting taken care of hadn't often involved sex.

Mike thanked them over and over again for the shoes and socks. They couldn't find him a place to shower in the hospital but he smelled much better after they threw away the old shoes.

Mike had described to Nurse Poole the classic symptoms of the onset of AIDS. He was clearly at risk for *pneumocystis* pneumonia, so he was given a follow-up appointment for April 26. He didn't keep it. In the meantime, his lab reports came back. Ironically, it was fortunate that Mike tested positive for syphilis—since he had a venereal disease, Kevin Burke was able to use the health department's sexually transmitted diseases unit to locate him. Kevin gave the unit a list of places where he thought Mike might be camping out and described the tent and the sleeping bag he'd given Mike—out of his own basement.

Health department workers found Mike at the AIDS/ARC vigil. Since October 1985, a group of people with

AIDS or AIDS-Related Complex and their sympathizers had been holding a sit-in in front of the old federal building to dramatize the need for more adequate federal aid and research. Mike had been sleeping there. It was safe.

Upset about having a venereal disease, Mike returned to Ward 86 on May 8. He felt much better and thanked Nurse Poole lavishly for the Acyclovir, which had cleared up his herpes. He complained about itching and appeared to have scabies. But the most arresting fact of his visit was that somehow, in the few intervening days, Mike had found a protector—a middle-aged, respectably dressed man whom he brought with him and introduced as his lover. Nurse Poole discussed safe sex practices with Mike, who didn't seem to understand exactly how AIDS can be transmitted.*

Mike had lost weight since his first visit. His cough was worse and he was running a 101-degree fever. On May 12, he was given a gallium scan and this lung X-ray, together with an examination of his sputum, confirmed the preliminary diagnosis of *pneumocystis carinii* pneumonia. He was admitted to the hospital for treatment on May 14. Mike had AIDS.

Even in the absence of *pneumocystis*, Mike soon might have been diagnosed with AIDS anyway. The definition of AIDS had been expanded by the Centers for Disease Control in 1985 to cover AIDS-associated opportunistic infections other than *pneumocystis* and non-Hodgkins

*Possibly, Mike had been living in a fog, but well into the epidemic, the exact definition of "safe sex"—beyond utter chastity—continued to remain vague in the minds of many. Although AIDS was a public health emergency, there weren't many mayors or even heads of health departments who were willing to go on TV and discuss "safe sex." AIDS had been declared the federal government's number one health priority, but in 1986 the president of the United States had not yet uttered the word "AIDS" in public. In many cities the media were reluctant to publish graphic guidelines. As for public education efforts aimed at drug addicts, the message was simple but the means of getting it to the people shooting up in alleys and abandoned apartments were pitifully few.

lymphoma—with the additional confirmation of a positive HIV antibody test. Mike, it developed, also had cryptococcus neoformans, a parasitic infection on the C.D.C.'s new list.

Mike was very ill. He was treated with Dapsone and Trimethoprim for 12 days but reacted badly to them, so his doctors switched him to intravenous Pentamidine for the balance of 21 days. Mike was lucky—the worst thing he developed as a result of treatment was a bad rash. These drugs are commonly used to combat *pneumocystis* and some of their possible side effects include: kidney damage, depression, loss of appetite, abdominal pain, hepatitis, diarrhea, headache, neuritis, insomnia, apathy, fever, chills, rash, light sensitivity, mouth pain, nausea and vomiting, low blood sugar, drop in blood pressure, pancreatitis, decrease in white blood cell and platelet count, and liver inflammation.

Mike sustained a high fever and this troubled his doctors. A new X-ray revealed nodules in the upper lobe of his left lung. Although he'd been cured of *pneumocystis*, Mike was also infected with cryptococcus. On June 6, he was placed on Amphotericin-B drug therapy. When he suffered from rigors and chills as a result, he was given premedication via the intravenous insertion of a Hickman's catheter on June 13. A "pocket" staph infection developed along the intravenous line and only cleared up after the catheter was removed a month later.

As a result of taking Amphotericin-B, Mike also suffered mild kidney failure and other minor side effects. During the course of continued hospitalization, he was given Clindamycin as a precaution against infectious toxoplasmosis. Since he had chronic oral thrush, or candidiasis, he was given Ketoconazole.

Mike had a painful but relatively benign infection of the lymph nodes. He complained of weakness and pain in his legs—tacit evidence of peripheral neuropathy, neural damage that is often a direct result of HIV infection.

During his stay at San Francisco General, doctors noticed as well what was obviously a Kaposi's sarcoma lesion on Mike's hard palate.

On May 16, Mike applied for Social Security disability payments.*

On June 6, he was given a lymph node biopsy at 2 p.m. and a CAT scan at 4.

On June 7, he was given a spinal tap at 9 a.m.

On June 9, he was given a bronchoscopy at 11 a.m.

By the middle of June, Mike was feeling much better and didn't require acute care. But he was still too sick to be discharged into what the social workers call "a marginal living situation," so on June 19, he was transferred to a chronic-care facility, the Garden Sullivan Hospital of the Pacific Medical Center.

In 1986 there were perhaps 3,000 homeless people in San Francisco and, in spite of the efforts of local private-sector agencies like the Shanti Foundation, a disproportionate number of them had become homeless because they had AIDS. It was, nevertheless, the unspoken policy of the mayor's office not to place people with AIDS in hotels along with other homeless people—so Mike and those like him were, as they say, "warehoused" in hospitals.

On June 22, after he'd settled into Garden Sullivan, Mike left the hospital on a day pass. He went to Macy's and bought a stereo-cassette player—a volunteer at San Francisco General had given him some gospel tapes but he hadn't been able to play them. Then he went to the Emporium and bought a datebook.

Mike's datebook is a small three-ring binder with a

---

*Once Mike was certified disabled by the Social Security Administration, he would get Medicaid as a matter of course. Without an officially sanctioned disability, it can take up to two years to qualify for Medicaid. And applicants have to "spend down"—that is, divest themselves of most assets—before Medicaid will step in to cover the enormous medical costs that accompany prolonged hospitalization. Mike had nothing to spend.

turquoise plastic cover. It contains a 1986 calendar, plastic pockets for credit cards and photos, 5 by 8-inch ruled sheets, and tabulated dividers. There are pages for addresses and phone numbers and for monthly, weekly, and daily planning. Since Mike died on September 25, the book is mostly blank.

Backdating entries, Mike began conscientiously to record the details of his hospitalization in neat, well-rounded handwriting. The datebook is evidence that he was attempting to come to terms with his experience and exert some control.

Some of the entries are poignant. *Very good and beautiful day for a Sunday,* he wrote on June 22. *Good to get out of for awhile. Feel great today!* The next day he wrote, *Today Dr. Fritz said that I may be able to get out in a week or two. Hopefully everything will go alright. Can't wait till that day comes!* On June 25, *Remember: Go easy and slow! Don't Rush Yourself.*

On June 29, Gay Pride Day, *10—Went to Parade / 11—Was supposed to meet Gary (no show) / 3—Came back and had a fever for the evening.*

A few friends, only identified by their first names, drift in and out of the pages of Mike's datebook—perhaps Mike's "lover" is one of those who seem to have dropped by the wayside when he was in the hospital. What's especially remarkable, however, is that at some point during June, Mike's father, whom he hadn't seen for at least eight years, flew out from Denver. Mike was eagerly anticipating his father's visit. And yet he didn't record it in his book.

3. THEY MADE SOME MISTAKE

What did she know about AIDS? There was a little boy in Indiana they wouldn't let back in school because he had AIDS. Frantic AIDS patients were turning to religion, positive thinking, kooky diets, mystery drugs, grasping at straws. Rock stars were making videos to raise money for AIDS. It was like everything else on TV—you tuned it out. Rock Hudson died and they said it was AIDS. He flew to Paris but he died anyway. A big movie star could die of AIDS but she never connected it with her son.

It was one of Mike's cruel jokes.

Then one night, her daughter Mary called.

"Mom, I don't know whether to tell you or not, but Dad told me to tell you—" Mary was in touch with Mrs. Rocha's ex-husband. Even though he lived just a few blocks away, Mrs. Rocha never talked to him. "Mike called him and he's really sick."

Her son always turned to his father first.

"Mom, I think Mike has AIDS."

This was like a big bell tolling. So he wasn't joking when he called in March.

"That can't be true."

"They told him," Mary said. "He had the test and everything."

"They made some mistake."

She refused to believe it. But then her ex-husband flew to San Francisco to see for himself and when he returned he called her.

"Nellie, our son is real sick," he said.

"What's wrong with him?"

"I don't know, but I wouldn't go out there if I was you."

"Why?"

"He doesn't want you to go out there."

"Where is he? What's the name of the hospital he's in?"

"He doesn't want to have anything to do with you. That's what he said."

Her ex-husband wouldn't give her the name of the hospital. She had to get it from Mary. Mary had talked to her brother. Mike was in San Francisco General Hospital. When Mrs. Rocha reached him there he said it was true.

"I have AIDS." Her son's voice was weak.

It was as if he reached through the phone and pulled her into another world.

"I want to go out to see you."

"No, I don't want you to come. I told you a million times I don't want anything to do with you."

"Whether you like it or not, I'm gonna come anyway."

It wasn't so simple. It took a long time. First she had to scrape up the money. Her husband said, How do I know you don't just want to take a vacation? She told him, I won't take a cent from you. Anyway, at that time he was only bringing home about $600 a month. She wasn't working herself. She didn't have any saved. And Mike argued with her. He said he wouldn't see her if she came. Then he didn't pick up his phone.

"I want to talk to my son."

"He has had pneumonia and his condition is stable," was all the hospital switchboard would say.

"But I'm his mother."

"I have no way of knowing that, ma'am."

She tried to find out who his doctors were. She called and called. All she got was the runaround. Finally she reached Mike again.

She could tell her son was afraid.

"I'm going to die, Mom."

He'd threatened suicide over the phone before. But this was different.

"Mike, do you want to come home?"

There was a silence, then he said, "No, Dad don't want me."

"What do you mean?"

"Dad told me not to go back home."

This was the father who always favored him, in whose eyes he could never do any wrong. This was the father.

"Do you want to come home?" she repeated.

"He told me you were going to call me and pressure me to go back home."

"Forget your father," she said, angry. "Mike, I don't want to pressure you. You don't have to come back if you don't want to but I'm coming out there."

He didn't answer.

"Mike?"

"Let me think about it."

On July 27, 1986, Manuella Rocha flew from Denver to San Francisco to bring Mike home. Some of her friends told her not to do it. They said everybody was going to get AIDS. Her own husband had said, I understand, you have to bring your son home, but by the time she left things were so bad between them, she didn't know if he'd be there when she came back. She told her husband at the airport, If you're uncomfortable, just leave. I'm not going to turn my son away for you.

She still didn't believe it was AIDS. She thought if she could just get Mike home.

Even after he said he wanted to come home, no one was really sure he would. Mrs. Rocha's second son, Larry, and her daughter, Dolores, decided to fly with her to San Francisco, thinking this might even be good-bye. It was very confusing. No one was sure how sick Mike was. By this time he was in another hospital, but why? And then the doctors had called Mrs. Rocha's ex-husband, too—they said someone might have to make decisions for Mike. He had something and his mind wasn't always right. What if he started going downhill?

Who knew what to believe?

Mrs. Rocha just felt that if she could get Mike out of the hospital and home he'd be okay.

She knew—they get all kinds of things and they die. In the two months since the news, Mrs. Rocha had read everything she could get her hands on about AIDS. She'd once worked as a housekeeper at the hospital in Greeley but that was the full extent of her medical knowledge. If she was going to take care of her son, she needed to know more. She called the hospital and they transferred her to the hospice for dying people and a girl, a nurse, came out to talk to her—Mrs. Rocha still didn't believe it then.

The hospice nurse gave Mrs. Rocha lots of literature to read and the number of this other nurse in Fort Collins who got her in touch with these people in Denver—the Colorado AIDS Project. This AIDS Project had a group for parents who had children with AIDS and the kindly nurse in Fort Collins even volunteered to drive Mrs. Rocha down to Denver for a meeting.

So one evening in June, Mrs. Rocha went to Denver in a car with three strangers and attended a meeting in a church where people sat around in a circle on folding chairs and talked about their sons who had AIDS. She didn't say anything. She just listened. Some of these parents' children had died. Some parents could cope with it, some couldn't. They were taking it, they said, one day at a time.

Some of the parents were mad at their kids. *Why did he do this? Why didn't he take care of himself? Didn't he know this could happen?* Some of them, like her, felt guilty. *If I'd done things different maybe this wouldn't have happened.*

She sat there in shock. She was numb. She thought, This isn't happening, this is happening to someone else.

She didn't say anything. She left in shock. She didn't know what she'd expected—maybe that they were going to say, It's going to be okay, they get better, they get well.

But she went back the next month. Without this group, she saw, she might go off the deep end.

The Mike in the bed was so changed. He was so sick. His features had changed a lot. He had lost a lot of hair—maybe he had lost a lot of hair because he was 29 already but it also was coming out in little clumps. Mike was so thin. When she hugged him she felt his bones.

Mike was so happy. He wanted to leave that same day but they had to make reservations for the plane to take them back. The Cancer Society had a room at the fanciest hotel in San Francisco all ready for them. Mike wanted to show them the city.

July 28 / 7—Woke up with toothache.

Mike didn't want them to come with him to have his tooth pulled, so the next day Mrs. Rocha and the kids did some sightseeing. They went to Fisherman's Wharf. They bought some souvenirs—T-shirts and stuff. That afternoon, they returned to the hospital and talked to Mike's doctor and the social worker, who seemed quite enthused. They said that with proper diet Mike might live two more years. Mrs. Rocha was overjoyed.

They had dinner with Mike off trays in the dining room there. Back in his room, they had a serious conversation.

"Mom, I've thought about what might happen, and what if I can't think for myself. I don't want any respirators or things like that. Will you sign a paper with me saying you won't let them do that?"*

She said yes, though she didn't want to think about that now. Everything was going so well. But then they got in an argument.

"I'm looking at your clothes, Mike. Don't you have no shoes or anything? Don't you want some clothes?"

"No, Ma, I'll do with what I have."

"Oh, Mike, you at least need a pair of tennies to go back home. Why don't you give me some money and I'll buy you some clothes before we leave?"

"Forget it, Ma."

So he wasn't so changed—he was paying for his plane ticket but he wanted to hold onto the rest of the money from his first social security check.

"Mike," she said, "you know this money you got out of the hospital safe today, we're going to need it when we get back, for your medications. We have no other way of getting your medications."

Mike turned his face away. "That's not my problem," he said.

"You're the one with the sickness," she said. "You're the one who's sick. I don't have the money for it. I'm willing to help you but you have to help me, too."

It was a few hundred dollars and he kept it close to his vest.

8—Went to sleep!

---

*At San Francisco General and Garden Sullivan, Mike was designated a "full code"—if he were dying, the staff would make every effort to save his life. In California, he gave his mother power of attorney to reject extraordinary measures in the event that he couldn't make decisions for himself. Therefore, during his last hospital stay, Mike was a "no code" and was allowed to die quietly and without intervention.

*   *   *

That next day, the hospital had all the papers ready
and Mike was discharged. He had a terry-cloth robe and
slippers that had been given to him by the San Francisco
gay bar owners. He had his datebook with some papers
and get-well cards stuffed into it. He had a pair of jeans
and some T-shirts and a new stereo-cassette player he
had never taken out of the box. He had all the materials
to make a hooked rug with a teddy bear in it. He left
some tapes and gay magazines behind.

Mike was so happy to be out of the hospital after so
many weeks. He wanted to show them parts of the city
he'd lived in for over two years. But as soon as they
took him out of the hospital, he turned a grayish
color.

"I wanted to take you out to eat, Mom."

"Mike, why don't we just go to the airport?"

Arrive airport check bag (very tired)

Their plane landed in Denver about 11. They got home
to Greeley an hour later to an apartment Mike never
knew, but he was home. Mrs. Rocha's husband was there.
All the kids were there but Rudy. Rudy was in Nebraska
but he sent his brother a letter. Everyone hugged Mike
because Mrs. Rocha had talked to them in advance and
told them there was nothing to be afraid of and they were
not to be ashamed, he was sick and needed their support.
They all sat up late talking. Mike was so happy to be
home.

Very tired / Hurray!

There was so much to do. When the lease on the place
they were living in ran out at the end of the week, they
moved to a two-bedroom apartment Mrs. Rocha had found
in a big old hip-roofed brick house so Mike could have a
room of his own—she told the landlady Mike had cancer.
The nurses came out from the hospice and brought sheets
and pads and all the things an invalid needs. They got

Mike settled into his new room. He was already gaining weight. She took him to the doctor and the doctor said he looked pretty good. She had hope.

Feel real good / home in Colo

4. WHAT'S PAST IS PAST

That first week they got to know each other again.
They went for a walk or a ride in the car, they sat
and talked, they went shopping or to get an ice cream.
Mike went to his nieces' softball game. His brother Larry
took him to the park. Mrs. Rocha drove him to K-Mart
and they bought a needlepoint set, a paint set to paint on
cloth, a cross-stitch set and a woodburning set. They
thought they might do some of this together but, as it
turned out, they never did any of it.

She thought they should clear the air, but Mike wanted
to put the past behind him. "What's past is past," he kept
saying. In San Francisco, he had said—

"Mom, I want to say something—I'm sorry for whatever I said or whatever I did. Sometimes I didn't know
what I was saying or doing."

"That's fine," she said. "Don't worry about it."

He had said over the phone from the hospital—

"I don't want to bring up the past. Let it be past. I
know I'm going to die and I want to go home."

Of his past gay life, Mike only said, "I was lonely and
lost then." Mrs. Rocha had met two boys, lovers, through
her group in Denver. One of them had AIDS and they

sent Mike a nice letter with a Polaroid picture enclosed of them together but he wasn't interested in making friends.

"I don't want to have anything to do with any more gay guys," he said. "I don't want to have any feelings for them. I thought I had friends but I lost them because of this disease. If I get better, I want to live a different kind of life."

"What kind of life?" she asked.

"I want to be able to take care of myself and live on my own."

She said, Well maybe you will be able to, but at the same time she knew Mike might die. She wanted Mike to make it right with his sisters and brothers before he did. She wanted him to make it right with his father. When he didn't call his dad, she said he must call. His father wasn't a well man. He had heart trouble. He'd quit drinking. His son should show some respect. So she knew Mike went to see his dad but not when. She didn't pry. One day Mike brought it up himself.

"You know, I didn't think you would ever want me back in your house again."

"Well," she said, "you were mistaken all along."

"I guess I was. I thought my father was the one who understood me. It wasn't so. My dad's a cop-out. It took me all these years to understand what my dad really is. You never said anything bad about my dad."

"No. He is your dad."

"And I knew why you divorced him only I didn't. I had my dad on a pedestal but it wasn't so. On my part—I don't know about the other kids but I wanted to treat you the way my dad did. I wanted to beat the shit out of you."

It hurt but she wasn't surprised to hear him say this. "And what did you gain from it?" she asked.

"Nothing. Dad didn't even want me to come back."

Before she went out to get Mike in San Francisco, Mrs. Rocha called the welfare office and they said Mike would be given Medicaid. He was already on Medicaid in California. So that next Monday, she took Mike over to the welfare building to apply.

They sat in the waiting room for half an hour. Mike was restless because his ass hurt so from the herpes he could never completely get rid of. Right now, aside from all his other medications, he needed medicine for the herpes. He was in pain. He kept standing up then sitting down then standing up. Finally, they were told they could go in and see Ms. Smith now.

They went in and said hello and sat down. Ms. Smith looked at the papers. "What can I do for you?" she asked.

"My son has AIDS and he needs to get on Medicaid," Mrs. Rocha said.

Ms. Smith put her head down.

"He just came home from San Francisco. I called a few weeks ago. I talked to this other lady, I forget her name, and she said to talk to you."

Ms. Smith didn't look up, she asked some questions about Mike's financial situation and how long he'd been in Greeley, and Mike answered, but she kept her eyes on the papers with her hand on her head.

At length, she said, "So you want Medicaid but he's not a resident of Colorado."

"He is now," Mrs. Rocha said. "He was born in Colorado," she added. "There's his birth certificate, a copy I got last month. It's an official copy."

"You know, I can approve or deny anything I want," Ms. Smith said.

Mrs. Rocha didn't understand. "Well, he needs Medicaid now, today."

Ms. Smith looked up from her desk and said, "You don't tell me what you need, I'll tell you what I can give you."

There was a silence. The two women glared at each other.

"Let's go, Mom," Mike said.

"You can go to the car and lay down if you need to," Mrs. Rocha told her son quietly.

"Let's just go."

"I'll be right back," Ms. Smith said, and she left.

They sat there.

Mrs. Rocha had never asked for welfare in her life. Since her kids were older, she'd always worked for a living. The truth was, she didn't know anything about welfare. They had told her in her group Mike should apply. She wondered if this woman knew she didn't know anything about welfare and was just talking through the side of her mouth.

This Ms. Smith was gone a long time. She came in then went right back out again. When she came back and sat down and started shuffling papers, Mrs. Rocha said, "Would you please hurry up? My son is not feeling well and he can't sit here all day waiting for you to get done."

Ms. Smith's lips were, by now, set in a line. She had Mike sign a bunch of papers.

"You know," she said to Mrs. Rocha, "if something happens, you're responsible."

"What do you mean?" Mrs. Rocha asked.

"It'll be in your shoes."

"He's signing the papers. I'm not. He's responsible for himself. He's a man now. He's a grown man. I'm not going to be responsible for anything."

Mike didn't say anything. He just signed the papers.

Mrs. Rocha asked, "How much will I be allowed for taking care of him?"

"What do you mean? He's your son. You don't get anything for taking care of him."

"I don't?" Mrs. Rocha was stunned. "Then how am I going to take care of him?"

"I have no idea."

"Then you'd better find somebody else to take care of him," Mrs. Rocha said, really heating up now, "and pay them, if I'm not allowed to take care of him. What about food stamps?" Mrs. Rocha asked. "Is he entitled to food stamps?"

"No." Ms. Smith spoke as if her patience were being sorely tried. "He is not entitled to food stamps. I don't think you understand."

"Well, why not?"

"Technically, he's not entitled to anything."

"What do you mean?"

Ms. Smith sighed and explained as she would to a child. "I'm going to give you these papers. You're going to take them downtown to the Social Security office to see if he can get SSI. Once SSI approves him, if they do, then you come back here."

"And what are we going to do in the meantime?" Mrs. Rocha demanded. "He needs his medication. Something has to be done because I don't have the money to buy his medication. How is he going to get his medications?"

"Look, there is nothing—the same way he's going to eat, I guess. How are you going to feed him?"

"Let's go, Mom," Mike said.

"It's none of your goddamn business how I'm going to feed him," Mrs. Rocha said. "I'm not asking you to feed him. All I want is medication for him because he needs it. He needs his medical for the hospital and all these other costs."

"Did any of this occur to you before you brought him back from San Francisco?"

Mrs. Rocha realized—this lady was afraid.

"Why didn't you leave him in San Francisco?"

"He's my son," Mrs. Rocha said. She spelled it out for Ms. Smith just the way Ms. Smith had spelled it out for her. "I couldn't leave him out in San Francisco. He's maybe dying. What would you do if it was your son?"

"I probably would have left him out there where he could get help."

"Mom, let's go."

Mrs. Rocha told Mike to go out to the car and lie down and when he left she turned to Ms. Smith and said, "Lady, let's step outside and I'll slap your face."

"Don't you threaten me."

"Now you look here, you're going to help me one way or the other," Mrs. Rocha said. "But I am not going to kiss your ass for a dime."

"And you look here," Ms. Smith said. "We are not responsible for your son. If SSI doesn't approve him, we can't do anything. Nothing."

Mrs. Rocha exploded. "Well why the hell are we talking here, then? I'm just wasting my time, is that what you're saying? And my son is sick and he needs to get home and I need to go home to take care of him." She could have wept. "Oh, just go to hell. Forget it." And she walked out.

When they got home she called the doctor and the doctor told her not to worry about it, he'd call up welfare and get a voucher for her for the drugs. When she worried aloud about the bills, he said, "Don't worry about it. Just don't sign anything. Somewhere down the line, they'll have to pay for it whether they like it or not. You have enough problems as it is." When she called welfare, Ms. Smith wouldn't talk to her but she went down and picked up the voucher from the receptionist and she never had to see Ms. Smith ever again.

The Social Security office was easier—thank God, downtown they took his papers and did the rest over the phone.

Her husband kept scrubbing the bathtub on his knees on the bathroom floor.

"Why did you do that? I just cleaned it."

"I wanted a bath."

"I told you, I just cleaned it. I just changed the towels."

But her husband kept scrubbing.

"I explained to you didn't I?"

Her husband wasn't a drinker but the first week Mike

was home he came home drunk every night. Once he was so drunk, he came home and went into the bathroom and passed out.

"You don't have any respect," she told him. "You don't have any respect for the dying."

She knew it was the AIDS. He said he was all right about it but what would you think if you saw a man turn into a drunk right before your very eyes, just like that?

"Look, if you can't handle this, get out," she said to him when Mike was out of earshot. "If you don't get out, I'm going to throw you out. I have enough problems as it is," she said. "I don't need to deal with this shit."

So her husband quit drinking. But he was still scrubbing the bathtub, changing the towels.*

"Well what do you think Mom? I'll probably be moving out of here pretty soon, on my own, get a job and be by myself, huh?"

---

*There have been no documented cases of casual, or household, transmission of the HIV virus, even where family members shared toothbrushes and otherwise lived together in circumstances with a high degree of physical intimacy. A tiny percentage of health-care workers have acquired the virus through their jobs; a handful of AIDS cases have been reported where workers were infected through needle pricks or, without observing standard precautions, had prolonged contact with HIV-infected blood and/or had a wound or other avenue to the circulatory system exposed to it.

5. IF THAT TIME CAME

About an hour's drive north of Denver on the South
Platte River, Greeley has been an important agricultural center since the middle of the 19th century, when it
was named after the same Eastern newspaper editor who
advised—Go west, young man. Depending on who's talking, Greeley is either a small city or a large town. Laid out
along City Beautiful lines, it boasts broad tree-lined streets,
a large city park, and the neoclassical porticoes of the
University of Northern Colorado. Downtown has pretty
well been superseded by the commercial strip, which has
its due complement of fast-food and auto franchises.

Local crops have long been sugar beets and grains but,
as everywhere, the small family farms are dying or dead.
Until not too long ago, this part of Colorado from the air
looked like a patchwork quilt or straw matting or crude
parquet wormy with gullies and creeks. In winter, the
fallow fields lay below like white table napkins, creased,
unfolded. There was something human-scaled and even
feudal about the landscape. But on high-tech farms today, the fields are watered and fed by rotating pipes on
wheels, so in some places it looks as if a prodigious stack
of phonograph records has been strewn across the plains.

To an outsider driving along Highway 85 from Denver, this country can seem relentlessly bleak. Once the land yielded up sod houses. Now it's dotted with silos, broken-down farmhouses, oil pumpers, cottonwoods lifting limbs like arthritic fingers to the sky. Ruled off by straight-edge roads, bisected by the interstate—like a zipper or an appendix scar—the landscape looks hard, flat, and unforgiving.

To the west, the earth swells, skews, bucks, and collapses against the feet of the Rockies. Seen from Greeley and the little town of Kersey nearby, where Mike grew up, the mountains don't seem quite part of the natural order of things. There's something abrupt and arbitrary about their appearance on the horizon. Even on days flooded with brilliant sunshine, clouds pile up along the shoulders of the mountains, white clouds, rolling in across the continental divide, unreal looking, like surf in slow motion.

In spite of his initial optimism, a little over a week after he arrived in Greeley, Mike had to be admitted to the hospital he was born in. His physician was William Jennings, a hematologist-oncologist at Weld County Hospital who also served as medical director of the hospice attached to the Northern Colorado Medical Center. By the summer of 1986, Dr. Jennings had treated fewer than four AIDS patients in a semirural practice that could hardly have seemed more remote from San Francisco and Ward 86—or even from Denver and Denver General Hospital.

Most of the 245 AIDS cases tabulated in Colorado thus far—the year before, 1985, the number had stood at about half that—had been counted in Denver. For most of its histroy, Denver maintained its identity as a raunchy, devil-may-care cow town. Now it was an enormous, sprawling city of some 1.5 million, many of them new residents drawn by the mild climate and generally high standard of living. Gay men were hardly oblivious to the allure of

Denver and the population included as many as 90,000 of them.

Denver's cosmopolitanism notwithstanding, Colorado is a politically conservative state. Quarantine of people with AIDS was seriously considered there and, by law, the names of HIV-positive individuals are on file with the health department. The fact that rates of HIV infection continued to be disproportionately low in the state was not, however, entirely due to the conservative social climate. Rather, it was due to the efforts of a few individuals who had heard the alarm bell in the early 1980s, set up the Colorado AIDS Project, and hastened to educate the state's gay men that waves of infection spreading across the country threatened to engulf them.

When he was admitted to the hospital on August 9, Mike was suffering from fever, confusion, and diarrhea. In his initial examination eight days before, Dr. Jennings had seen in Mike a man in declining health. This impression was confirmed by the discharge report from Garden Sullivan Hospital—which amounted to a concise chronicle of AIDS-related debilitation. When he'd first examined Mike, Dr. Jennings noted continuing evidence of cryptoplasmosis leading to sepsis and pulmonary involvement.

Mike was destined to be one of the 14,345 AIDS-related deaths reported in the U.S. by the end of September. Although the actual cause of his death would remain a mystery—his family refused to permit an autopsy—it clearly involved progressive respiratory failure presaged, of course, by the *pneumocystis* pneumonia and cryptococcus he'd been treated for in San Francisco. Finally, something prevented the transfer of oxygen from the air in Mike's lungs to his blood. His pulmonary system would continue to deteriorate through another course of treatment for *pneumocystis* and beyond.

In his initial examination, Dr. Jennings had found continuing evidence of all the complaints Mike had reported in San Francisco—painful enlarged lymph nodes, chronic rectal venereal warts, chronic rectal herpes, thrush, and anemia. Mike complained of worsening pain in his legs and his Kaposi's sarcoma lesions had proliferated—he now had four to five purplish, bruiselike cancers on his hard palate, two to five on his trunk, two to three on his right flank, and one on his left forearm.

Dr. Jennings also noticed a variable degree of alertness in Mike, and this, perhaps more than any of Mike's other symptoms, convinced the doctor that Mike belonged in the hospital. Dr. Jennings ordered a spinal tap, thinking Mike might have an infection of the central nervous system, but nothing was found.

Perhaps surprisingly, considering all Mike was enduring, he continued to exhibit no symptoms of manic-depressive disease. All the same, Dr. Jennings was confronted with a different patient from the one who presented himself at Ward 86 in May. Lauren Poole met a waiflike survivor with all his wits about him. Dr. Jennings met a sad and angry man who talked in a flat voice and exhibited no sense of humor. Mike didn't strike the doctor—who routinely dealt with cancer patients—as a person who wanted to live.

The doctor said they just wanted to do some tests but Mrs. Rocha knew. They got things then they died. She knew now, they'd been fooling themselves. They'd heard what they wanted to hear in San Francisco. She'd felt so good when he started to put on some weight but the fact was, in every other way Mike had been going downhill since he got out of the hospital in San Francisco. He was sick on the plane.

Now she realized what was happening to Mike. She could see it in his eyes. There was a faraway look in his eyes now. His eyes were glassy. She'd seen the same look in her brother's eyes before he died. She'd seen it in her father's eyes when they put him in the nursing home.

When she pressed Dr. Jennings, he didn't say much,

just that he couldn't predict how long Mike would live. "I don't want to tell you that he's going to last this long or that long, because that only complicates the situation." She knew, sometimes they struggle on and on.

Dr. Jennings told her he thought Mike's mental attitude was knocking him down. She agreed with this. But what good would it do to tell Mike his mental attitude was important, give him some kind of pep talk? If she could see death in her son's eyes, he could read what was on her mind, too. Even if she wanted to, she couldn't lie to Mike. He'd laugh in her face.

Dr. Jennings said that after a point the idea was to keep Mike comfortable. Yes, that's what they wanted done, she replied, no respirators or any machines if it came to that, if that time came.

He went in on a Saturday and they let him out on Tuesday. He announced he was going to California.

"I might want to go back to San Francisco."

"What do you want to do that for?"

"This is going to be too much trouble for you, to deal with this."

"We'll deal with it together. Is there anything you want to talk about?"

"No."

But she could see how troubled he was. He didn't talk. He didn't watch TV. He didn't read. He just lay in bed looking at the ceiling. When she entered the room, he would close his eyes and pretend to be asleep.

He wouldn't take a bath. She let a couple of days pass before she said, "Mike, you have to get up and take a shower."

"I don't feel like it."

So a few more days went by and she told him, "Mike you have to get up and take a shower or let me help you take a bath."

"Bug off," he said. "I don't care if I die dirty or not. Just leave me alone. Quit bugging me."

She sat down on the end of his bed.

"Mike, do you really believe you have two years to live?"

"No, I'm not gonna live that long," he said. "I don't want to anyway. I knew a guy in the hospital in San Francisco, they told him one month, the next month he was gone. Once they diagnose your AIDS, you're gonna die, Mom. I know that. You're not gonna last long. I want to die, too. I'm tired of living this way. I don't want to hassle with it anymore. But I'm afraid to die till I make things right with God. I fucked up my life. I would like a priest."

So she called Our Lady of Peace and the priest said, "Father Urban lives right across the alley from you." So Father Urban came and talked to Mike and gave him Holy Communion. Mike was very happy. Father Urban was very nice. He said he'd be back. But he never came back—she'd see him outside when she was hanging the wash out on the line and he wouldn't look her in the eye. Then one day, Father Urban ran into Mrs. Rocha's friend Shirley on the street and asked her if she would mind giving Mike Holy Communion. Shirley was taken aback. She asked Father Urban, Wasn't it up to him to do that? Maybe Father Urban was afraid after all. Whatever. He never came again, and Mike said, "To hell with him."

One day she saw Mike take papers out of his datebook and rip them into tiny pieces and throw them in the trash.

The pain and weakness in Mike's legs got worse. Larry would come and take his brother out in the wheelchair, wheel him to the park. Mike was unsteady on his feet and often Mrs. Rocha's husband would have to help him move from here to there. Yes, her husband was good to Mike. He took him to the flea market in the wheelchair.

When she was out, he stayed with Mike and warmed up his food for him. Other times, Shirley, who had known Mike since he was little, since Kersey, sat with him.

The first week he was home, lots of relatives came to welcome Mike back. She had told them all he had AIDS and some of them were scared but came anyway. One of Mrs. Rocha's sisters told her, "The gays are going to go to hell," but her older brother said, "Things happen, who knows why?"

Now Mike's sisters and brothers still came to see him and he would talk to them but if anyone else came he complained, "Mom, I wish these people wouldn't come over. They freak me out. It's like they're coming to see some kind of side show."

Anyway, the curious would come once to see for themselves a man with AIDS and then not come back. Friends who had known Mike from childhood wouldn't touch him. They would stand at the foot of his bed and talk from a distance.

Mrs. Rocha's friend Lucy came but couldn't sit down. She would sit down then stand up.

"Lucy, what's wrong with you, you're so nervous."

"Oh, I just hate to see people sick," Lucy said.

"You want a Coke or some pop or something?"

"Yeah, sure—don't put it in a glass," Lucy added.

Some people never came. Mrs. Rocha's brother's wife never came. When Mrs. Rocha saw her in the Safeway, Tommy's wife said, "I would come down but I don't want to take this sickness to my family."

(Tommy's wife wept at Mike's rosary and said how sorry she was. A week after Mike's death, she appeared at Mrs. Rocha's door early in the morning. As Mrs. Rocha looked on, her sister-in-law washed all the dirty dishes, stripped the beds and made them up fresh, dusted, vacuumed, scrubbed, cleaned, and tidied the apartment.)

Mrs. Rocha's friend Irene never came. After her divorce, Mrs. Rocha lived with Irene for three months, they were so close. But in June, when they were having coffee and Mrs. Rocha told Irene she was bringing Mike home, Irene said, "Oh, I wouldn't do that."

"Why?"

"We're all going to get AIDS then."

"If you'd let me explain what AIDS is, maybe you'll feel different about it," Mrs. Rocha suggested.

"No—I don't want to know."

It had just been a few weeks, but Mike was now a complete invalid. He was gaunt. His eyes were deep in his face. He had an invalid's slight tremor. He had an invalid's problem with time. His memory was going, too. He didn't always remember which pills he had taken when. He was on painkillers and Mrs. Rocha knew that if he wasn't watched he would overdose. He hoarded his pills just as he'd always hoarded everything—little things when he was a kid, nothings that he kept to himself, money if he ever had any.

It became routine. Sometimes twice a week, hospice volunteers would bring bedding and pads and other supplies. The nurse would come and take his temperature, check his blood pressure, and treat his herpes—it was bleeding all the time. The men who brought the oxygen wouldn't come at first but the boss made them come back.

One day Mike might get up and have diarrhea all day. He tried to keep himself clean. He would put the pads in trash bags. But some days he would mess the bed two or three times a day. There was a washer in the basement and Mrs. Rocha used it sometimes two or three times a day. When it got too hard to get the blood and shit out of the sheets, she would just throw them away. The hospice kept bringing new sheets.

Before her husband came home from work, at 5, Mrs. Rocha would have supper alone with Mike. Sometimes it would sit all right with him. Sometimes he would throw up right away, sometimes later. One night she went into

his room. His breathing was ragged. It frightened her.
She lifted him up and he threw up all over her, head to
toe. She cleaned herself off. She cleaned him up. She
changed the bedding. She cleaned up the rug.

When she bathed him, his hair came out in her fingers.

He was restless at night. He slept during the day. He
would turn on the TV then fall asleep. He would stay up
all night. Her bed was on the other side of the wall from
his. She would hear him moving around.

When she got up to check on him, he would say,
"Mom, go to bed."

One night she sat on the edge of his bed and talked to
him.

"What's bothering you, Mike?"

"Nothing. I just can't sleep."

"No, what's wrong?"

"I don't want to go to sleep. I'm afraid I'm going to
die."

"But you could die during the day, too."

"But you're here then," he said. "I worry about death a
lot. It frightens me, to die."

What could she say?

"It frightens me, too. We're both scared of it."

She'd go outside to hang up the wash and she'd only be
gone five, ten minutes. He'd say, "Gee, you were gone so
long." When she had to go out and clean house in the
mornings because they needed the money, Mike would
call her wherever she was. "Aren't you done yet?" he
would ask.

One day she saw him tear up a letter he had written to
Terry and Gerry, the lovers. He tore it up into little
pieces.

He was jaundiced. His feet were swollen. His speech
was slurred now. His mind was not right. He was having
trouble thinking.

6. GOING TO GO HOME

I took him to the emergency room about 1 or 2 a.m. and he had a lot of diarrhea and they put him on this stretcher and he was just full of diarrhea and they left him there for about half an hour. Finally, I told a nurse, 'Why the hell don't you change him? How would you like to lay in a pile of shit?' is what I told her. He had taken an overdose of morphine and painkiller so they gave him something to counteract the medication, I don't know what. He was in a lot of pain. He was just there screaming. He was in this diarrhea and they put a fan there to take away the smell. I told her, 'Instead of getting rid of all that shit? What the hell is a fan going to do?' He was in the emergency room. It was just a big room where they have curtains. Finally they cleaned him up and put him in his room.

When the time came for him to go home, the doctor and the hospice nurse and I talked about it. They wanted him to make a contract to see if he would exercise, get out of bed—get up at a certain time in the morning, take a shower, comb his hair, go for a walk, or whatever. And they told him that if he didn't agree to sign this contract that they wouldn't let him come home, he would have to stay in the hospital. They thought if they made this contract with him it would bring him out of the depression he was in, because he was real depressed—in order to get him to want to live.

So we made up this contract and he signed it and he was really mad at me.

When he went back home that last time he said, 'I just want to die. I'm not going to try anymore. Not you or Dr. Jennings, not nobody is going to make me eat or do what they want if I don't want to do it.'

He said he just signed the contract so he could come home, it was not that he was going to keep it.

I told him, 'Mike, I don't know what to do with you. You can't lay in bed and not take a bath. You have an odor anyway as it is.'

I don't know, it's a certain odor that they have. I don't know what it is. They get this odor like death.

And he had gotten this one check and I told him, 'You have to help us with some of these bills we're behind on.' But he wasn't about to part with that $500. I said, 'You're going to have to pay some rent, help us pay the rent and at least buy extras, things that you want to eat—maybe you'll feel better.'

And he said no.

And I said, 'I'll buy you some clothes'—because he didn't have any clothes and stuff. Finally he agreed that he should have clothes. I got him some underwear and some socks, T-shirts.

He wouldn't eat or drink no more or nothing. He wanted to go to the hospital in Denver real bad. So the doctor finally got him to Denver. It took about three days.

Mike said he was going to go to Denver and he was going to die. He said, 'I know, I have seen AIDS patients die.' He said, 'I'll have a lot of pain and they'll have to give me morphine to keep me comfortable and then I'll go into a coma and then I'll die.' He didn't want to be at home.

On September 18, after a week in Weld County General Hospital and three days at home, Mike was taken to Colorado General Hospital in Denver for bronchopulmonary lavage—literally, his lungs were flushed. The procedure had to be done in Denver because the hospital in Greeley wasn't fully equipped for it.

During Mike's second stay at Weld County, Dr. Jennings had made an empirical diagnosis of *pneumocystis* pneumonia and treated him accordingly. The doctors in Denver found no residual evidence of *pneumocystis* and no definitive reason for Mike's continuing pulmonary decline. Finally, they told Mike and his family what they already knew—that he didn't have much more time to live. Mike's reaction was stoic.

Mrs. Rocha shuttled back and forth from Greeley to Denver. The Colorado AIDS Project helped her with money for gas and a new friend from the parents' group offered her a bed on those nights when she didn't return home. At the hospital's suggestion, she began to look into the possibility of hospice care should Mike improve enough to be released.

Mike was no longer afraid to be alone. In the evenings, he'd say, "Go, Mom, go home."

"I don't want to go."

When she called on the phone, he'd say, "Don't bother me, Mom, I want to rest."

On September 24, six days after he entered Colorado General, Mike's spirits lifted. "I'm happy now," he said. "I'm going to go home."

"What do you mean, you're going to go home?"

"Ma, it's okay, don't worry."

That day, he was given doses of liquid morphine at 3 p.m., 6, 7, and 10. He looked so well, Mrs. Rocha wondered if he was going to live longer than the doctors expected. He looked better than any time since his first week home in Colorado.

He'd refused to see a priest for many days running, but that evening he acquiesced. The priest gave him last rites.

Mike was happy. He ate a little food. He talked on the phone.

Mrs. Rocha's parents' group was meeting that night. "I'm going to go to the meeting then I'll come back."

"Mom, don't come back till the morning."

But she got out of the meeting at 10 and went by the hospital with her friend anyway.

Mike was awake. The little cup of morphine was at his bedside. "What are you two doing here?" he asked. "Bar-hopping tonight?"

"Ohhh, yes." The two women laughed.

Mrs. Rocha noticed, Mike had hung up the phone crosswise—he'd left the receiver off the hook.

"How come you have the phone like that?"

"I was just talking to Larry. I want to rest now."

"Did you call your dad?"

"No, I didn't call Dad. Larry called and I talked to him. Look, why don't you go home. There's no need for you to be here all night. Go home now and don't come too early in morning."

She hugged him and he hugged her. She cried.

Mike died the next day, September 25, 1986, at 9 a.m. When Mrs. Rocha arrived at the hospital early that morning, he was in a coma. He looked peaceful. His forehead was unlined. When he died, his mother was holding his hand.

Do you know what we're like, Chicanos? The same town, the same block, your mom and dad, your sisters and brothers—we stick together. You grow up with your family and all your relatives and even if you leave home, home is always home, no matter what. My kids, we may fight, have arguments, whatever, but there's a home here. Your folks are your folks, that's all.

All those years I was hoping he would come back to me. No matter what he was or what he did—that was his life to live, he chose to live that way. I hoped he would come back to me.

At the beginning of October 1986, Mike's disability check arrived in the mail. Mrs. Rocha called the Social

Security office and was told to go ahead and cash it to pay some of her bills. Subsequently, though, she got a letter asking her to come into the office, where she was informed she had to give the money back. It was $533. She paid off her debt in installments.

1987

And the Lord said unto Satan, Whence comest thou? Then Satan answered the Lord, and said, From going to and fro in the earth, and from walking up and down in it.

—*The Book of Job*

LINCOLN HOSPITAL,
THE SOUTH BRONX

Barely half an hour from midtown Manhattan, the big red-brick hospital is located in the South Bronx, a world apart. The hospital was founded in 1839 by a group of white women to provide relief for aged blacks, many of whom had been slaves. The hospital's coat of arms reads— Health, Dignity, Compassion.

The present, thoroughly modern hospital building cost $250 million and was opened in 1976. A part of the municipal hospital system, it was built to accommodate 750 beds and currently operates with 539. The hospital's occupancy rate is 97 percent, the highest in the system.

In early 1987, the Democratic party power establishment in the Bronx is in turmoil following a series of scandals involving bribe taking and political corruption. Since the upper echelons of the hospital administration tend to get filled with patronage appointees, this disarray has extended to the hospital. The most recent administrator resigned amidst allegations that he'd received kickbacks from hospital hiring practices.

The organization of the hospital is compartmentalized and the member-states don't always communicate. Apart from administrative departments, there are departments for adult psychiatry, medicine, gynecology/urology, surgery/

neurosurgery, plastic surgery, oral surgery, orthopedics, obstetrics, and pediatrics. The hospital's emergency department handles over 220,000 patient visits a year; its outpatient clinic, over 500,000. The hospital transfuses nearly 7,000 units of blood annually. Support services include chaplains, patient advocates, social workers, and volunteers. The hospital has a barber shop, a beautician, a playroom, a coffee shop, and a gift shop.

The hospital stands on East 149th Street beside commuter railroad tracks. To reach it on foot from the Grand Concourse, you walk across a bridge over the tracks. There is a chain-link fence along the bridge to keep people from jumping off it or throwing things onto the trains. Even during cold winter days, street peddlers hang brightly colored skirts on the fence and set up tables sheltered from the biting wind in the lee of semi trailers the post office parks along the street. The peddlers sell fruits and vegetables, flowers, sweaters, jackets, handbags, jeans, cosmetics, incense and ointments, framed prints—glossy photos of sports cars, exotic flowers, women in skin-tight pants and spiked heels—even bed pillows. You have to keep walking, past the hospital, up a long, long block to Third Avenue, to buy drugs.

1. THE LIST

February 17, 1987. It's Tuesday after the long weekend and no one wants to be back at work, so the meeting starts a little late. This morning three people in white lab coats sit at the table. A reporter is also here, so everyone's a little nervous. It isn't often that someone who isn't manifestly ill comes into this closed world from the outside.

The hospital AIDS team meets in this room every Tuesday morning, almost without fail, to review the inpatient list. In the beginning of the epidemic, when there were only one or two people with acquired immune deficiency syndrome in the hospital, there wasn't any need to consult on a regular basis. But by this time last year, on any given week, there were a dozen or more AIDS patients in the hospital in addition to many more being seen in the outpatient clinic, so the team was formed to advocate for them. Now there are routinely more than two dozen names on the weekly inpatient list and the epidemic shows no signs of peaking—not here at least, among the poorest of the poor. Here whole families have died of AIDS.

The team meets in the Infection Control unit on the seventh floor in a large room with four desks that are usually occupied by nurses. There's a bulletin board covered with greeting cards, printed notices, and a bumper sticker that reads "Infection Control Nurses Get The Bugs." Like many of the staff rooms in the hospital, this one feels claustrophobic. There are only three portholelike windows high up on the wall and they can't be opened. Little light penetrates. It could easily be dark outside. It is 9:40 a.m.

Judith Lieberman, clinical director of the Infectious Disease service, leads the meeting. The others sitting at the table are B.C. Gerais, a pharmacological psychiatrist, and Robert Carter, a social worker. The team is short two members. The nurse assigned to it full time is on leave and, because the pay is low relative to that at a voluntary hospital, no one has yet answered the advertisement placed in the papers some time ago for an outreach social worker. The Catholic chaplain, Sister Fran Whelan, is a sixth, *ad hoc* member of the team. Sr. Fran has been working with AIDS patients since the beginning of the epidemic—in fact, she was the only one visiting them for some time. Sr. Fran does a lot of bereavement counseling.

Head down, elbows on the table, wearing a button that reads WASH YOUR HANDS, Dr. Lieberman plows through the patient list, taking each in turn, reciting facts and figures, exhibiting uncanny if not total recall of the circumstances of each case. Dr. Gerais—a petite, irrepressible woman, called Babe by her friends—sits next to her making notes on three-by-five cards imprinted with patients' names and hospital registration numbers.

Today the list consists of 23 names with chart numbers, admission dates, room numbers, and diagnoses, recorded on a form in neat black Palmer penmanship and photocopied for the team early this morning.

Almost invariably, the column headed "Diag." on the

list simply reads AIDS, but in a few instances it reads R/o AIDS because some patients are waiting to find out if AIDS can be ruled out in their case. The majority of AIDS patients on the list have *pneumocystis carinii* pneumonia— and for some reason, February is a peak month for pneumonia—and/or opportunistic infections like crypto-coccal meningitis, centomegalovirus, and toxoplasmosis. These are AIDS-related infections that sometimes went unrecognized and undiagnosed a few years ago—patients were dying so quickly—but were included in the revised 1985 Centers for Disease Control definition of AIDS. Dementia, an illness similar to Alzheimer's disease, and emaciation, a wasting away, are now considered by doc-tors virtually to define AIDS as well.*

There are no transfusion-related or hemophiliac cases on the list—few, if any, are ever seen at this hospital. And only a small minority of patients in this hospital displays the skin cancer, Kaposi's sarcoma, that was at first a primary indicator of AIDS. Kaposi's sarcoma is still most often seen in homosexual males, and now—for some reason—less frequently at that.

Most of the people with AIDS in this hospital have a history of intravenous drug abuse. The staff calls them IVDAs. These patients got the so-called AIDS virus from sharing contaminated needles. Other AIDS patients here were their sexual partners or children. They acquired their HIV—for human immunodeficiency virus—infection via sexual intercourse, in the womb, or during birth.

*These diseases, with a confirming HIV-positive antibody test, were subse quently added to the official definition of AIDS effective September 1, 1987. In one stroke, then, the number of people recognized as having AIDS in the U.S. increased by 20 percent—to more than 41,000. Anticipating this statistical leap, the federal bureaucracy ruled in June that people with AIDS suffering from dementia or emaciation did not automatically qualify for Social Security disability insurance, although anyone with AIDS had before. Explaining the rationale behind this decision, one official of the Social Security Administration was quoted in *The New York Times* as saying, "They may be dying, but they might not be disabled." The Government eventually reversed its ruling.

Four patients who have been diagnosed with AIDS-Related Complex, or ARC, have been placed on the list, yet the list doesn't represent the total number of AIDS-related cases in the hospital. Between 70,000 and 97,000 New Yorkers have ARC, over seven times more than have AIDS, but six years into the epidemic, ARC still constitutes a vast, shaded area of diagnosis.

People who never reach the point of an AIDS diagnosis can die from diseases associated with HIV infection anyway. Endocarditis, for instance, is a heart disease often seen in drug addicts. A full 90 percent of endocarditis patients in this hospital also have candidiasis, or oral thrush, a good indication that they are immune suppressed. If those patients were added to this morning's list, there would be twice as many people on it. Even in 1987, the full ramifications of HIV infection are not yet fully appreciated. For example, three of the ARC patients on the list today have TB—epidemiologists speculate that HIV infection accounts for the first rise in the incidence of tuberculosis since 1953. Chronic renal failure is also emerging as another, more subtle byproduct of AIDS.

The list has all the ingredients of a soap opera:

One woman with AIDS was discharged over the weekend because hospital police found vials of crack on her.

One man with AIDS can no longer recognize his sister.

One woman with AIDS who is ready to go home can't because her daughters, addicts, threatened to harm the home-care attendant when she came to introduce herself.

One man with AIDS walks around the ward, wheeling his intravenous stand along with him, socks crammed with cash.

Dr. Lieberman plows through the list.

Not infrequently Dr. Lieberman looks exhausted, and today is no exception. For one thing, she's due at the dentist's for root canal work. But if you were to ask her directly, Dr. Lieberman would willingly admit that the job is getting to her, too.

Dr. Lieberman is under a lot of stress and much of it is simply due to "the system"—the great, amorphous, many-tentacled system that holds her hostage along with everyone else in the hospital. Like everyone who works inside the system, Dr. Lieberman is constantly frustrated by it and fighting against it. The system sees to it that patients' charts disappear, that specimens are lost on the way to the lab, that sometimes obtaining a necessary service or commodity from another part of the hospital depends mainly on the goodwill—and skill—of individuals.

Mr. Husseni, for example, is recovering from *pneumocystis* pneumonia, but lately he's been exhibiting certain personality changes. The other day, Dr. Lieberman was able to persuade him that the diagnostic spinal tap he had long refused to permit wouldn't hurt too much. She promised him it would be easy but it wasn't. It was very difficult. His spine was clenched tight and the interns just rammed the needle in through the vertebrae. Mr. Husseni screamed in agony throughout. As an intern herself, Dr. Lieberman developed a shell, and she moves about the hospital inside it, but she still can't stand to hear a patient scream.

The system can be almost diabolically unresponsive to patients with AIDS. Technicians are preparing to perform a crucial liver biopsy. The patient coughs. They refuse to stay in the room. The distraught 11-year-old daughter of a dying woman can't get counseling. The child psychiatry department hasn't yet perfected its policy on children of patients with AIDS.

Sometimes you can only laugh.

Of course AIDS is not the only fatal disease in the hospital. Many patients die here of cancer or liver disease from alcoholism. But Dr. Lieberman did not train to be an oncologist treating cancer patients. In fact, she deliberately chose infectious diseases as a specialty because she wanted to be able to make people well. She certainly did not expect to see people in her care die in such numbers—only three other city hospitals have more AIDS patients than this one.

In addition to her hospitalized patients, Dr. Lieberman sees outpatients in the weekly parasitology clinic—no one wants to call it the AIDS clinic—so each week she's in contact with lots of people who have AIDS. Dr. Lieberman is in her thirties. Since people with AIDS are on the average from 29 to 35 years old, many of her patients are her contemporaries. Just as she does, they have family concerns, concerns about money, surviving in New York. Some of them, she knows, are felons on the street. But the hospital is a leveler. Naked, sitting on a table in the examining room, under the white glare of fluorescent lights, waiting for the doctor, perhaps fearful, a man or woman is most vulnerable, most human.

Dr. Lieberman likes her patients almost without exception. They aren't objects to her. They're people. She gets to know each one of them intimately. She also must daily live with the fact that she will usher many of them with AIDS in and out of the hospital time and time again—until the end comes.

The problem of burnout among doctors, nurses, and other health-care workers in the hospital who have to face a seemingly endless procession of deaths from AIDS is not often confronted directly. Like everyone here who treats patients with AIDS, Dr. Lieberman has learned to rely on sharing her feelings of grief and anger with colleagues. Sometimes, in order to continue functioning, she must simply set feelings aside, like a letter from the I.R.S. you put off opening. If she allowed herself to cry as often as she felt like crying, she would be crying a lot of the time.

Dr. Lieberman routinely has success treating the opportunistic infections that initially accompany AIDS, with medications like Amphotericin-B, Septra, and Pentamidine. She can buy time for patients. The experimental drug AZT, much in the news at present, has given doctors new hope. Though toxic, it seems to arrest the spread of the HIV virus and has clearly shown promise among a few categories of AIDS patients. Nevertheless, Dr. Lieberman knows that she will probably continue to be a relatively helpless witness to her patients' decline and demise for many years to come.

There are no routine AIDS cases. Today, for instance, the list is full of anomalies. One man on the list will die this afternoon, presumably of an infection generally considered treatable nowadays. In the absence of this underlying, incurable immune deficiency, such cases might have represented unusual, even stimulating challenges to Dr. Lieberman and her colleagues—including the young residents under her supervision who earnestly sweat through Socratic instruction over a stack of pink patient status sheets with her during weekly rounds. But in the shadow of AIDS, this reading of the weekly list sometimes resembles a macabre bookkeeping chore more than it does the practice of medicine.

So Dr. Lieberman plods on.

Part of her problem is semantic. What should she call an alien, untoward abscess that has emerged out of a wasted body like a special effect in the movies? Resorting to euphemisms is an inescapable tic. This morning she calls it "something weird." *General deterioration, fever of unknown origin, empirical diagnosis.*

Dr. Gerais is at least free of that burden. Dr. Gerais knows psychosis when she sees it and her pharamacopia is ample. With a single injection Dr. Gerais can knit up the raveled sleeve of care until it unravels again. Dr. Gerais must only listen. Last weekend, for instance, she spent an hour listening to Mr. Cintron, who she discovered liked best to be called Roberta. Mr. Cintron was in the early stages of a sex-change when he came down with AIDS. He is very weak but his spirit is strong. When Dr. Gerais asked him if he had a lover, he snapped back, "I can't be in love now, my machine is out of order." Mr.

Cintron's family—his mother, his brothers and sisters—
has rallied around him and they all visit him in his room.
He is "she" to them, too. In his cross-dressing days, Mr.
Cintron was a prostitute. "Name it and I did it," he told
Dr. Gerais last weekend. Probably, this is how he con-
tracted the HIV virus, and possibly passed it on to others.

In some ways, Dr. Gerais has a pleasant enough job.
Her patients are often anxious, for example, that she like
them, because many of them are drug addicts accustomed to getting what they need through manipulation,
not the kindness of strangers. Typically, they are demanding, immature, and needy. Many of them are clever,
witty, verbally adept people who are only too pleased to
wisk her along in a breakneck, sometimes electrifying
circuit through the corridors of their psyches. Of course
Dr. Gerais is also accustomed to listening to long, tedious,
self-justifying monologues riddled with delusion. Mrs.
Thomas, for example, the mother rendered homeless by
her addict daughters, presents herself as a frail wraith at
the mercy of circumstances beyond her control. Actually,
she's a strong matriarch and a longtime drug abuser who,
though desperately ill, disappeared from the hospital last
December and returned, high, hours later, saying she'd
been out doing some Christmas shopping.

Sitting across the table from Dr. Gerais, Mr. Carter
keeps his place on the list with the point of his pen.
Owlish behind eyeglasses, Mr. Carter reads the paper
systematically, front to back, every day. He begins with
the national news on the subway in the morning and
finishes with the arts pages at home. No less methodical
about his work, he has already been through the activity
log this morning to update his records—he keeps entries
on each patient in a big black three-ring binder and
weeds out the discharged or dead every few months.
Slightly stooped, world-weary, Mr. Carter has worked at
the hospital a year and a half now, always with AIDS
patients. Before coming here, he was a psychologist in

private practice. But he felt isolated, and friends of his
had died of AIDS, so he sought out this job. He doesn't
make an effort to hide it, but not many people here know
that Mr. Carter is a Jesuit priest. Social work is just the
most recent in a series of callings. For Mr. Carter, "the
list" is perhaps the latest of God's more inscrutable texts.

Mr. Carter runs an outpatient group during clinic on
Wednesday afternoons and an inpatient group on Fri-
days. He visits patients. But much of his time is spent on
the phone, making referrals and trying to secure services
for his clients. More than once, he's at last located help
for a patient only to find he's no longer able to locate the
patient.

Mr. Carter, too, has listened to his share of pathetic
testimonials. As he well knows—since it's his often futile
task to "follow" patients into the real world—addiction in
one form or another permeates this part of the city, the
community devastated by it, the hospital itself. Addict
patients keep leaving against medical advice, to get a fix.
Sometimes they argue, sometimes they just walk out, sometimes they check back in. Continuity of treatment is difficult if not impossible to maintain. Invariably, some patients
who have been detoxified in the hospital go back to their
habit on the street, where suicidal gestures are commonplace anyway. Some patients who are discharged from
the hospital never appear in the outpatient clinic for
follow-up care and reappear only in the emergency room.

Mr. Carter has listened to his share of deluded resolu-
tions. No one, including him, completely trusts the addicts in their midst, and with reason. Hated in the
community with a contempt bred of abject familiarity and
fear, addicts in the hospital are a category apart from the
other patients—in their own eyes, in the eyes of the staff,
even in the eyes of their loved ones. And an addict with
AIDS, even one flat on his or her back in the hospital, is
somehow more contemptible than the neighborhood junkie
shooting up downstairs in the hall. This is partly because

addicts have passed on AIDS to their wives, husbands, and children—however innocently—and partly because, in this religiously conservative, overwhelmingly black and Hispanic community, AIDS is still thought of as a disease confined to homosexuals.

It isn't, of course. Thus far there have been 31,000-plus cases of AIDS in the U.S. since the Centers for Disease control started counting in 1981 and blacks and Hispanics made up a disproportionate number of them. Although blacks and Hispanics comprise 20 percent of the U.S. population, 39 percent of those with AIDS nationwide now are members of those two minorities. Blacks alone make up 12 percent of the United States population but account for 25 percent of all AIDS cases.

Nine out of ten children with AIDS in the United States belong to a minority. According to the Centers for Disease Control, a black woman in 1987 is thirteen times more likely to be at risk of infection with the HIV virus than a white woman, a Hispanic woman eleven times more likely.

In New York City, black people make up 31 percent of AIDS cases, Hispanics 23 percent. But many black and Hispanic leaders are still reluctant to discuss AIDS. Some fear a backlash against minorities already victimized by discrimination and they don't want to become identified with the disease. In addition, financial and other resources are scarce in their communities. Minority groups would have to struggle hard to match the social and support services marshaled by the gay community—which, like the Gay Men's Health Crisis itself, is certainly not confined to but is largely defined by white, middle-class men.*

---

*The full extent of the epidemic among minorities in New York City will come into sharper focus later this year when the health department releases almost comically precise estimates of the numbers and kinds of people it figures are infected with the HIV virus. These will include 200,785 whites, 118,171 blacks, and 95,838 Hispanics.

The health department will estimate that there are 366,616 men and 48,178 women in the city infected with the virus—212,500 homosexual males, 37,500 bisexual males, 111,375 heterosexual men who use drugs intravenously, 30,000 women who use drugs intravenously, and 15,678 women who have been infected by male sex partners.

Intravenous drug abusers themselves account for fully 75 percent of AIDS patients in New York's municipal hospitals. They make up almost 90 percent of so-called heterosexual-contact cases in the city. Around 37 percent of AIDS cases citywide now involve addicts and their heterosexual sex partners and/or their children. Moreover, new data suggest that AIDS among addicts has been underreported by as much as fifty percent. A recent review of deaths and illnesses among intravenous drug users in the city in 1985 indicates that typically where a death certificate specified endocarditis, pneumonia, or another illness that commonly accompanies immune deficiency, the actual underlying cause of death was AIDS. Numerous cases in this statistical population might have been incorrectly categorized.

As if responding to potent prejudices, the city's social service system—inflexible, inefficient, worn out, reflecting a society weary of palliatives—has moved late to address the special problems addiction presents in relation to the epidemic. As it is with numbers of sexually active gay men transmitting the virus through intercourse, the numbers of addicts sharing dirty needles add up to a staggering rate of infection. There are over 200,000 drug addicts in New York City. That figure doesn't include people who have been off intravenous drugs for as long as five years and might just be starting to exhibit symptoms of infection. The patients in the hospital today are the advance guard of a veritable army of HIV-positive potential victims of AIDS.

Public health education has come too little and too late for thousands of addicts. At present, the surgeon general of the United States seems to stand alone in the top echelons of the federal government in insisting that AIDS be treated as a medical problem requiring explicit education to prevent it, not moral nostrums. Mass public education on the efficacy of condoms has been on government's back burner for years now. The propriety of network TV commercials for condoms is still being debated. In the meantime, increased media attention to AIDS again seems to have set off shock waves of fear, even among those least at risk in the heterosexual population. In the midst of this emotional, politically charged climate, public education aimed at addicts is not receiving the attention it merits—attention is diverted from it by squabbles over sex education in the schools.

Merely warning a drug abuser once or twice about the dangers of sharing needles is, in any case, a feeble weapon against the spread of AIDS. Addicts are by definition an impulsive group of people who ritually and for a variety of reasons share needles and syringes. The idea of dispensing sterile "works" to addicts is seductive in its simplicity, but in 1987, it is considered politically unfeasible, if not counterproductive from a public health standpoint.

"Just say no," the slogan goes. But not many alternatives to addiction are available to drug abusers in New York. Drug rehabilitation programs are few and have long waiting lists for admission.

According to some estimates, between 1981 and 1985, mortality among IV drug abusers in the city increased an average of 30 percent. Given this, the sluggish response of government to the plight of addicts might be seen as some kind of "final solution to the addict problem" —although moral theologians would stop short of any comparison of the AIDS epidemic with the Holocaust, advocates for the welfare of addicted people aren't so reluctant to make this equation. Since some of the AIDS-related maladies drug users suffer from especially still aren't, as of February 1987, included in the definition of AIDS, they don't officially have AIDS. They thus aren't even eligible to receive Social Security disability payments.

As Mr. Carter is only too aware, his patients aren't the only ones in the hospital at the mercy of the sometimes

capricious vagaries of the social service system. He became a dependent of it himself the day he signed on at
the hospital. He can't help patients without it. But with its
endless succession of forms, coupons, and Alice-in-
Wonderland regulations, the Department of Social Services functions like a Ruritanian bureaucracy in wartime,
and Mr. Carter is sometimes relegated to stretcher bearer.

Today—again—he's going to try to get a wheelchair for
Armando Santiago.

The meeting ends at 11 a.m.—but not before Dr. Gerais
announces that she's tendered her resignation. When Dr.
Gerais was assigned full time to the AIDS service a few
weeks ago, she promptly had her office in the outpatient
clinic taken away. In fact, she came into work one day
and found someone else sitting at her desk. Now she has
no place to see patients or keep her records, and since no
office is forthcoming, she's going into private practice.
(True to her word, Dr. Gerais left the hospital a month
later.)

When Mr. Carter comes into the room, Carmen Baez is
scrubbing the rails of Mr. Santiago's bed with alcohol.
There is a pink "precaution" sheet posted on the door to
this room. Some nurses on the ninth floor put on a mask
before they go in. Nurse Baez isn't even wearing gloves.
The housekeeping staff is supposed to keep the room
clean. But Nurse Baez likes hands-on nursing. She likes
to do as much as possible for her patients.

Dressed in a blue paper hospital gown with a paper
sash at his waist, a brown knit cap perched on his head,
Mr. Santiago is sitting in a chair. Grey stubble lines his
jaw. When Mr. Carter comes into the room, Mr. Santiago's
face turns anxious.

Mr. Santiago has been in the hospital with toxoplasmosis, an infection that causes brain abscesses, since December 27. He's well enough to leave now. He is waiting for

his wife to come take him home but his wife hasn't even visited since last week.

When Mr. Santiago came to the hospital, he was incoherent. On his first visit, Mr. Carter couldn't tell what language Mr. Santiago was speaking. Then he didn't talk for a week. Then gradually, he began speaking in Spanish. Then his wife showed up.

When Mr. Santiago's wife comes to the hospital she smells of alcohol. It's hard to get anything out of her. When she doesn't want to answer questions, she begins to speak in Spanish. Before he came to the hospital, Mr. Santiago was living alone in a rented room without heat or hot water and his welfare case had been closed. But now, his wife says, she's found an apartment for the two of them—although the last time Mr. Carter saw her she said she couldn't remember the address of the new apartment. It didn't have electricity, she said, but her brother was going to fix that.

Partly because he's been in bed since December, Mr. Santiago's muscles are atrophying and the people in Rehabilitation say he can't go home without a wheelchair. Since Mr. Santiago can't afford a wheelchair and hasn't yet qualified for Social Security disability payments, Mr. Carter has been trying to tap into a special fund for wheelchairs. The wheelchair hasn't come yet, but then neither has Mr. Santiago's wife.

When Mr. Carter sent a letter to Mr. Santiago's son at the address given to him by the son, it came back stamped "address not known."

Everyone's waiting for Mr. Santiago's wife to come take him home. No one knows how to reach her. No one knows her at the phone numbers she's given. Maybe she's wandering from place to place. For a while she visited her husband regularly and even helped him do the movements Rehab prescribed. But maybe it finally sank in, what her husband has.

"Has your wife come to see you?" Mr. Carter asks Mr. Santiago.

No, Mr. Santiago shakes his head.

"Do you remember what we talked about, about Coler Hospital? Maybe I can help you get into Coler Hospital," Mr. Carter says, speaking slowly and distinctly, "where they'll give you better care than we can."

Mr. Santiago looks uncomprehending.

"I'm still trying to get you the wheelchair," Mr. Carter says.

Nurse Baez gets up off her knees. "You mind if I say something, Mr. Carter? You know, he doesn't need a wheelchair. He can walk, can't you, Mr. Santiago? I wondered—he'd be sitting in the chair and I'd come back in and he'd be in bed. I asked him, How'd you do that? And he said, Walked. Come on, Mr. Santiago." Nurse Baez speaks to Mr. Santiago in Spanish.

She helps Mr. Santiago stand up. Since his limbs are emaciated, Mr. Santiago looks like a clothespin doll in the paper gown. Together they demonstrate—Mr. Santiago can walk.

"It's not good for them to sit in a wheelchair," Nurse Baez says. "Not if they can walk. I argue with the nurses, Don't put the side rails up because the man is gonna hurt himself because he can walk and he'll get out. Because he does."

Seated now, Mr. Santiago listens to Mr. Carter and Nurse Baez discuss his problem. His head swivels back and forth from one to the other. Looking up at them, his eyes are frightened, searching.

In the bed next to the door there is a big, heavy black man with a huge growth on the side of his face. He is brain dead, on a respirator. His heaving coal-colored chest and stomach are bared.

2. PEACE ON EARTH

E very time one of her patients leaves the hospital, Carmen Baez says, "I hope I never see you again." But half of the patients on her floor have AIDS and almost all of them return. Usually they die in the hospital.

These deaths are not easy. Nurse Baez gets involved with her patients. She makes it her business to know their business. They tell her their life stories. They look to her for emotional support. She has hugged them. She has kissed them. She has sat down and cried with them.

The hospital is trying out something new on Nurse Baez's unit—primary nursing. So she's been assigned approximately ten patients and acts as their advocate as well as their nurse. She doesn't just make their beds, take their vital signs, and then go onto someone else. She explains their medication to them, their disease, the process of the disease, its complications, follow-up checkups, and a lot more.

Nurse Baez always wanted to be a nurse. When she was little and someone asked her what she wanted to be, she would say, I want to be a nurse with 13 children. She would take off her dolls' clothes and examine the dolls, prodding them with her fingers. She would put pretend slings on her sisters' arms. When she went through a tomboy stage, she was always falling down but she always knew how to patch herself up. Her mother would say, Rub butter on it, but Carmen would argue that she knew something better. If someone got cut, she was never afraid to look at the blood.

Before Carmen ever went to nursing school, when her sister had her first baby, Carmen used to walk around holding him under her arm, like a football—this horrified her sister but later in school Carmen learned that's a perfectly good way to hold an infant. The first time the baby got a rash, Carmen went out and bought cornstarch. The rash went away. When the baby caught a cold, Carmen put him on her lap with his head down and tapped him. The congestion came out. There were a lot of things Carmen did right from instinct, without knowing they were right in advance.

Nurse Baez went into nursing late, at 26, when her second child was nine months old. Part of her training took place at this hospital. She came here for three years, off and on, and was hired when she graduated, almost exactly a year ago. Her first four months on the floor were like a crash course in suffering. Lots of patients died—that's the way it is in Medicine, as opposed to other departments. Each time a patient died, she wept. And yet in a curious way, Jimmy was the first patient who really got to her down deep. No one will reach down that deep again.

He wasn't even her patient. He belonged to another nurse. But she would see him.

It was hard to ignore him. He'd walk out of his room naked. He'd defecate all the way down the hall. Like one of her babies. He was 24 years old.

His name was Jimmy Sanchez and he was brought to the hospital at the end of May by his father. Carmen says that when he came in Jimmy had bruises and cuts all over his face and on his back. She says he was mad at his father for bringing him. She says he claimed that his father had drugged him and brought him to the hospital against his wishes. But Jimmy had been wandering the streets, his father said. He had to bring in Jimmy. They didn't know what to do with him at home anymore.

Jimmy's mother died when he was four. Soon after, his father, Daniel, married again, to an amiable woman named Laura. Laura raised Jimmy. Jimmy always called Laura "Mommy." He never called Daniel "Daddy" or "Dad" or even "Popi." He called him Daniel. When she saw Daniel embrace his children, Carmen says, it was not exactly the way you embrace your child. Something—some warmth, some lack of reserve—was missing.

Jimmy's family was religious and upstanding. Jimmy went to college. As soon as he could, he left home.

He found a lover, an older man, a black man who was married, and he moved to New Jersey to be near him. Jimmy got a job as a technician in a factory. He had an apartment and a car. He had his own life. All this hurt Daniel, who didn't understand his son.

There was anger there. But when Jimmy got sick, in January last year, he ran away from the hospital in New Jersey to come home to his father's house in the Bronx.

Jimmy was changed. He acted crazy. Then, too, he would wander off. He would fall down.

When Jimmy's father brought him in, he had *pneumocystis* pneumonia and subacute encephalopathy, also called "AIDS dementia." In his dementia, Jimmy regressed to an earlier age.

Nothing fazed him. The nurses would tell him, "Jimmy, you have no clothes on, you can't do that, go back to the room," and naked, Jimmy would stare at them as if asking why.

At first Carmen simply observed. But then she got more and more curious. Why was Jimmy acting this way? And something about Jimmy struck a chord in her. Jimmy yelled, Jimmy shit his pants, Jimmy was as demanding as any two-year-old. He was a problem child. The thing was, no one else seemed to see just that—Jimmy *was* a child. He was like a baby. Carmen had babies of her own. Carmen loved her babies. Jimmy struck that chord.

Jimmy was medicated but he was too ill—he was often intubated with intravenous lines—and too contagious to be on the psychiatric ward. But he was really too crazy to be on a regular floor. Jimmy was restless. When left unattended, he made a mess of his room. He would defecate and then smear it all over. And he liked to walk around the unit, naked, pestering the staff, fouling the floors. It was an impossible situation they just had to deal with—that there was no place for him, Jimmy, in the hospital. No wonder no one seemed to want to take care of him. But Carmen wanted to. Carmen felt a tug. So Carmen began asking if she could take care of Jimmy. It took a long time, but gradually, unofficially, Carmen became Jimmy's nurse.

Jimmy got better. His pneumonia cleared up. His madness progressed.

One day they found him dressing in his room. He said he was going to sign out. So they had to take away his clothes. When they did that, Jimmy was left with no personal possessions.

Sometimes they restrained Jimmy. Sometimes Carmen had to tie him to a chair with a bedsheet. She would position the chair in his room so he could watch TV or look out into the hall. Sometimes Jimmy seemed content to sit there in front of the little TV his parents brought him.* Other times, he'd cry out for Carmen as soon as she left the room—

"BAEZ!"

---

*Rules that are often ignored in the hospital include:
• No electrical appliances such as razors, personal TV sets, hair blowers, and radios—radios with headphones are particularly prized by patients.
• No visitors who are ill.
• No food or drink in the patients' rooms.
• No smoking in the patients' rooms or corridors.

Soon everyone got used to hearing Jimmy screaming Carmen's name at the top of his lungs. Only Carmen could calm him. No one else would do. If the doctors came to see Jimmy, they had to fetch Carmen before they could touch him. If he heard Carmen talking at the nurses' station, he'd call her away. Jimmy would yell so long and loud, the supervisors would make Carmen leave another patient to quiet him. "Go over there and tend your child," they'd say.

Jimmy was Carmen's baby. Because he could not be responsible for his bowels, she put paper diapers on him. Since he was always taking his clothes off, she put three or four gowns on him at a time. In the place of a pacifier, she rationed out cigarettes—in spite of his pulmonary condition, Jimmy smoked as many cigarettes as he could get his hands on. Jimmy was a cigarette-smoking, coffee-drinking, big bass-voiced baby about six feet tall.

No one wanted to take care of him. He was a nuisance to everybody. The only other person on the unit who could tolerate Jimmy was Louis, the housekeeping guy. Louis would talk to him in Spanish, bring him coffee, give him a cigarette, and watch over him while he smoked it. One day when Louis finished mopping his room, Jimmy turned his cup upside down and poured his diet supplement all over the floor.

"Jimmy! How can you do that? You just saw me mop the floor!"

"Good, now you can mop some more! You don't have to leave me alone!"

They got used to thinking of him as a child.

Jimmy was his adult self only once all the time that Carmen knew him. One day, about three weeks after he came to the hospital, when Carmen was tidying his room and they were talking, she asked him if he knew what he had.

"I don't know."

"You mean the doctors haven't explained your diagnosis?"

"No, why?"

"I just want to know, to see if you have any questions that I can answer."

Suddenly Jimmy was yelling. "I have AIDS! I'm gonna die! I'm gonna die!" He got distraught. "I don't wanna die, Ms. Baez! I don't wanna die!"

Oh, my God, Carmen thought, this is what's been bothering him. This is why he turned into a baby. She said, "Jimmy, we all have to die. That's something that's inevitable."

"But it's not my time now and I'm gonna die anyway."

Carmen's eyes filled with tears and she went to Jimmy and put her arms around him. She consoled him.

This was his one lucid moment. The psychiatrists had interviewed him and he could remember everything in his past—when he was a child, about his mother—everything up to a certain age, then he blanked out.

"BAEZ!"

He was her baby. Carmen found herself bringing him candy and cakes. At home she would talk about Jimmy. Her husband knew all about Jimmy. He would see Carmen pouring coffee into the thermos. "Oh, this is for Jimmy"—because Jimmy hated the coffee in the hospital, she made him Spanish coffee at home. And Carmen's husband would tell her, "You have another son, you know, on the job." "Yeah," I do, she would say. "You," he would tell her. "I don't know why you decided to go into nursing, sentimental as you are, emotional as you are. You're going to have a nervous breakdown."

At first Daniel was the only one who came to visit Jimmy, but eventually Carmen got to know the rest of Jimmy's family—Laura, his sisters. Sometimes Jimmy was withdrawn, blank, and apathetic, but not around his father. There was anger there.

Daniel didn't understand that his son had regressed

and kept demanding something Jimmy could not give him.

"You gotta stop talking so loud, Jimmy," he would say.

Or, "Jimmy, you have to eat all your food and be neat and stop all this nonsense" when Jimmy just could not do that.

"I don't want Daniel to visit me anymore," Jimmy would say to Carmen. "You tell them downstairs in Security not to let Daniel come up here anymore."

"Jimmy, that's your father. Don't you love him?"

"Yes, I love him."

"So why don't you want to see him?"

"He gets me so upset."

So Carmen talked to Daniel and told him to try not to expect too much of Jimmy. But it hurt Daniel, to see his son like that.

When Jimmy was well enough to go home, his family said they could not take him and that they were afraid for the children there. So Jimmy was put on the Alternate Level of Care list, which meant trying to place him in another facility, but he didn't leave 9-A alive.

Jimmy would wander around. Carmen kept layering him with gowns to keep him covered. He suffered from bouts of diarrhea, so Carmen kept diapering him and told him if he had to go to the bathroom please to let her know.

One day, unobserved, Jimmy went into the bathroom in front of the nurses' station. He took off the diapers and must have tried to sit down but he missed the toilet. When he tried to clean up the floor, he got it on the wall. When he tried to clean the wall, he smeared it all around. Silently, Jimmy padded out, leaving tracks down the hall, and returned to the nurses' bathroom with a bottle of iodine spray. Whoosh, whoosh—he sprayed the room with iodine.

"Jimmy, what are you doing?"

"Cleaning."

"My God, he used the toilet!" Nurse Taylor got hysterical. "We have to call housekeeping! My God, he used our toilet!"

"I'm sorry, I'm sorry," Jimmy was saying, but everyone was running around ignoring him.

"We have to do something about him," Nurse Taylor had once said, but Carmen just replied, "He's always tied down, let him walk."

While everyone was running around, Jimmy went to the activity board. He was erasing it. Carmen just sat there and watched him. He erased everything. Then he began writing.

"What are you doing now?" Nurse Taylor screamed at Jimmy.

Jimmy turned around and when he turned around they saw what he had written. It said PEACE ON EARTH.

"Peace on Earth, Nurse Taylor," he said. Then he went straight to his room.

"I want you to take me to the second floor."

"What for, Jimmy?"

"I'm going to apply for a job here in housekeeping."

"Jimmy, why?"

"Cause I want a job here. The hospital picnic is tomorrow, look, see? They're getting things ready." He pointed to the lawn outside the window, between the hospital and the parking lot. "Look, they're having a picnic and the only ones that can go are employees and I want to be an employee so I can go."

His lover came. His lover's wife came too, a very old woman. They owned buildings in the city and they came in to collect the rents. They had papers for Jimmy to sign. They wanted Jimmy to sign over his disability checks. There was a paper giving Jimmy's lover permission to take Jimmy's money out of the bank.

Later, Jimmy's sister screamed at him, "That faggot came over here, taking advantage of you, taking your money!"

Jimmy said, "But he doesn't do that. He's not taking advantage of me. He's trying to help me."

"Help you! He took your car, he won't let us go in your apartment and get your pictures or anything!"

From then on, the few times Jimmy's lover came, Carmen was standing right beside the bed.

She heard someone talking to Jimmy.

"You know what you have, right? You have AIDS and you're gonna die. How long is it that you have?"

"No no no," Jimmy was saying. "I'm not gonna die. Who told you that? Who said I had AIDS?"

It was Jimmy's stepbrother. They had grown up together. No one had seen him for months. He was dead drunk.

A hospital isn't a good place for someone with AIDS to be—they're exposed to all kinds of infections. And so it was with Jimmy. He got every little thing.

The diarrhea worsened. One day he started bleeding from his rectum.

The next morning, when Carmen came on at 7:30, she went to open Jimmy's door but one of the other nurses going off duty said, "No, he's sleeping, he just fell asleep. Don't wake him up, please, otherwise he's going to start yelling." So Carmen went about her rounds. At 8:15 she returned.

She opened the door. The room was full of shit and blood. Shit and huge clots of blood covered the floor. It covered the bed. Jimmy was naked. They'd strapped him to the bed by both wrists but somehow he'd managed to work one of the restraints loose. His body was twisted across the bed. Shit and blood were still pouring out of him. His feet were slipping and sliding in it.

"My God, how can they do something like this?"

Carmen ran to the door and called the head nurse. She snatched a gown up off the infection cart outside the door and pulled on gloves. She ran back to the bed and tried to prop Jimmy up.

"Oh, my God."

The head nurse came to the door and her face turned ashen.

Outside, Carmen put on a yellow surgical gown and booties over her shoes. She put on a surgical mop-cap. She went back into the room and laid absorbent blue pads all over the floor. She made a path through the shit and blood to the bathroom. She put Jimmy on the toilet.

While Jimmy sat on the toilet, she changed the bed. She turned the water on in the shower.

"Jimmy, you're going into the shower, let's go."

He didn't want to but she got him into the shower. "It hurts!" he complained. He was sitting on the floor of the shower and the water was striking his face. He tried to crawl out of the shower.

"No you don't."

Carmen got halfway into the shower with him. She took some of the soap from the dispenser—it smelled good. She washed his hair.

"Wash yourself."

But Jimmy refused.

"Okay, that's it, I gave you your chance," Carmen said. She got some pads and soaped them up and she began to scrub him all over. "What are you doing?" he squealed.

"I'm washing you. I'm cleaning this garbage off you."

"Okay," Jimmy said. "Just don't touch too low."

So she bathed him and dried him off and dressed him and got him back into bed. Louis came to clean up the room.

"Jimmy, you like to give me a lot of work, don't you?" Louis said.

"Yes!" Jimmy said. "Yes!"

*   *   *

Jimmy had multiple blood transfusions. He was bleeding and losing control utterly but the surgeons didn't
want to intervene. They came into the unit and put in
packing. Maybe their reasoning was that he had not far to
go.

Jimmy got *pneumocystis* pneumonia again. He wasn't
eating well. They were feeding him intravenously. Carmen kept bringing him Spanish coffee but he wouldn't
drink it. At the beginning of August he was put on the
critical list.

When Carmen came on the morning Jimmy died, she
went to his room. Laura was sleeping in a chair. She'd
been there all week. When Daniel came in with coffee,
they woke up Laura.

"Look," Carmen said, "you've been here all night. Why
don't you go home, take a bath or something, then come
back?" They tried to persuade Laura but she stayed on.
Finally, about ten, she went home.

Carmen told Daniel, "I have to go do my assignment. I
have work to do." Daniel was jumpy. He'd been there all
week, too. "If you need anything call me." She knew, the
slightest thing, he'd call. That's what he'd been doing all
week. She began her rounds.

He didn't call. He ran to her.

They rushed to Jimmy's room. He had such pain on his
face. He was white. He was gasping for air.

Her eyes filling with tears, Carmen looked at Daniel.

Jimmy was a "no-code"—no extraordinary measures,
no machines, no resuscitation.

Carmen wanted something to be done. She knew nothing could be done, but she didn't want to let go.

She ran and got the doctor and the head nurse. The
doctor came in and looked at Jimmy. Daniel was outside
in the hall, so after thinking a moment, the doctor said in
a low voice, "It's going to be a silent code." They would

try to keep Jimmy alive a bit longer but the code wouldn't be called through the loudspeaker.

They told Carmen to get the code cart. Her heart was pounding. She was trying to be strong. Outside the room, Daniel had a bewildered look on his face. She ran down the hall.

They had a new clerk at the nurses' station and when he saw Carmen getting the code cart he called the code over the loudspeaker before she could tell him it was silent.

"1269A."

Everyone came running.

Carmen wheeled the cart to Jimmy's room. The head nurse was standing outside the door. Daniel was standing there, stricken. Carmen opened up the cart.

One of the nurse's aides ran up saying, "The administrators' is on the phone. They want to know whether this is a code or not, or what's going on."

The head nurse stared into Daniel's eyes. "I cannot answer you with his father right in front of me," she said. "Please go away." She opened the door and Carmen wheeled the cart into the room.

They weren't doing anything.

The doctors were standing around the bed, talking quietly among themselves. It was supposed to be a no-code but because the father was there they made it a silent code but someone mixed it up and they called the code—

"What's going on? What are you going to do?" Carmen asked.

They didn't answer.

She pushed them away and stood over the bed and looked down at Jimmy. Tears were oozing out of his eyes. She took his hand.

"Do you know who this is?" she asked him.

Jimmy was fighting to breathe. "Of course I do."

"Who is it?"

"Baez."
Tears were falling from his eyes. Then he took his last
breath.

*I wouldn't go to the funeral because I don't go to funerals—I
mean the actual burial. I don't go to cemeteries, not even for my
own family. But I did go to the funeral parlor. I told my
husband, 'You have to take me because he's going to be there and
I promised Daniel I would go.' He said no. He was totally
against it. He said, 'I don't want to take you over there. You
have to be professional and separate the two things.' And I said,
'I can't because I wasn't only professional with Jimmy. I got
involved with him and out of courtesy to the family and just to
see him for the last time, take me to the funeral home.' So he took
me.*

*I decided to wear white. It wasn't my uniform. But Jimmy had
met me in white, always saw me in white, so I said, Let me go for
the last time and see him in white. It was the beginning of
August. I remember having my white sandals on.*

*So I went and my husband stayed outside with the children.
He knew it was something I had to do so he let me do it alone.
And I went inside and the family was there. Everybody was
sitting down. So I went in and I walked straight to the casket.*

I heard them say, There goes Jimmy's nurse.

*He looked so old. He didn't look like the Jimmy in the hospital.
When he died, he was white—you know, it was the look of death
on his face. But in the casket he was, like, purple. It wasn't the
same Jimmy. They'd combed his hair so he looked like Daniel a
lot at that point.*

*One of the daughters came up behind me and she hugged me
and she started crying on my shoulder. And I was pretty strong. I
didn't cry. I had already been to the hospital psychiatrist two or
three times so I'd gotten it out and I was able to be strong. First
of all, I didn't want to go back in the car and have the children
see me all upset. Then I knew that I couldn't break down because
Daniel and Laura would.*

I wasn't with them too long because I knew if I stayed too long it was gonna hit me and I was gonna start all over again so I stayed just for a few minutes.

It really took me a while to be able to walk onto the unit and not think of him and to be able to walk into that room and not think of him. It was totally another unit when I walked onto it and I didn't hear Jimmy say, Baez—you know, the way he used to yell out, bellow. He had such a deep voice. It took me a while to get over that.

Now I care for my patients and I'm human and whatever, but I don't let myself get as close as I did to Jimmy because I don't think I'd be able to go through the pain again. I don't like to see people die, but it's not like—you know, the pain. I pray when they die and I'm taking care of their body, wrapping it up. I pray to the Lord, take this soul with you, at least something has ended, which is what is important. But I try not to be so involved like I was with Jimmy.

About a month after Jimmy died, a young man came onto 9-A, feverish with a viral syndrome—not AIDS. He was 19.

"Hey, you knew my cousin," he told Carmen, "because he was your patient."

"Yeah? Who was your cousin?"

"Jimmy Sanchez."

She saw the resemblance there.

"Okay," Carmen said. "I have to ask you some questions for the admissions sheet. You do drugs?"

"Yes, I use drugs but my mother doesn't know so please don't tell her."

"Let me see your arms. I don't see any tracks."

"Every time I use it I'm careful. I try to do it in the same spot and I put creams on it so it won't get scabby."

"Do you know what your cousin died of?"

"Yeah, he died of AIDS."

"Don't you understand this is a good way of you getting it? If you share needles?"

"Yeah, yeah."

Carmen had another patient in an isolation room and he was dying of AIDS. He was in the last stages. He'd been an addict for 20 years. Carmen went to this man and told him, "I have a kid who's 19 and using drugs. He's being discharged today. This is not standard procedure at the hospital, but I'm taking it upon myself to ask your permission for him to come in and see you—see you the way you are now."

He looked at her, and he said yes.

So she persuaded Jimmy's cousin to go into the room and there was shock on his face because he knew the man in the bed. He had sold drugs to the man when he was healthy. Now he was in a hospital bed with tubes coming out of his chest, a skeleton with a cover on it.

They talked. Carmen sat down in a chair and waited for them to finish talking. And when they left the room Jimmy's cousin confessed that he was dying to leave the hospital and go into the streets and take another shot. But after seeing the man in there he swore he was going to think about it first.

She hasn't heard from Jimmy's cousin since. She wonders whether to believe him or not but she hasn't seen him back at the hospital.

3. A WALKING PLAGUE

February 18. This afternoon the downstairs corridors of the hospital are crowded with people—people loitering, people staggering, people searching, people passing through, people laughing, people eating, people drinking, people smoking, people staring, people dozing, people trying to squeeze by. There are people on crutches, people in wheelchairs, guards, nurses, cops, patients and their families. The corridors are crawling with a surging mass of people.

Perpetually, people are waiting. A long line runs around the corner and down the hall from the cashiers' windows. A long line snakes around roped stanchions in front of the pharmacy windows. In the outpatient waiting rooms people sit in rows of chairs. ("Patients aren't called patients for nothing," puns Mr. Carter.) In the halls and the waiting rooms, there are puddles of cola and coffee on the floor. Everywhere, there is an air of resignation and imminent alarm.

The corridors are full of noise. Everyone is talking. Lite F.M., piped in through ceiling speakers, is playing. Somewhere an elevator alarm bell rings unceasingly—its message goes unheeded as the elevator moves from floor

161

to floor. Someone is shouting into the receiver of a pay phone. Vending machine levers rebound with a clatter. The doors to the emergency room bang open.

Every year, over half a million outpatient visits are made to the hospital. This Wednesday afternoon, 28 outpatient clinics are being held here. These include gynecology, occupational therapy, dental services, neurology, urology, plastic surgery, and the weekly so-called parasitology clinic. Mr. Carter manages to commandeer an examining room for his outpatient group, which is composed of people who have already been in the hospital at least once with complications from AIDS or ARC.

This isn't how they told Mr. Carter to run a group in school. There aren't enough chairs, so someone perches on the lid of the trash can, someone else on the edge of the examining table. Others lean against the wall. Patients drift in. They're called out to see the doctor. The group is always liable to get evicted. Conversation is desultory. Mr. Carter doesn't lead the group. Nor does he contradict misguided or misinformed statements. He sits and listens. Now and then he encourages someone to talk. If people talk he can say he's had a good group.

Today before clinic he runs into Diego Ruiz and Alberto Flores in the hall, talking to Luis Alegria. As he promised he would last week, Mr. Ruiz—instantly Dino to everyone he meets—has brought a newsletter published by an organization called ADAPT. ADAPT stands for the Association for Drug Abuse Prevention and Treatment. The group is right now for drug abusers what the Gay Men's Health Crisis was for gay men at the beginning of the epidemic, six years ago. Dino and Mr. Flores follow Mr. Carter back to the examining room—Mr. Alegria, who says he's depressed and wants to be quiet, stays behind in the waiting room.

The health department estimates that over half of the addicts in New York City are infected with the HIV virus. Most of them are heterosexual. The Centers for Disease

Control says that fully 5 percent of heterosexual men ages 30 to 39 in New York are now infected. According to the ADAPT newsletter Dino brought with him, most of the 36,000 people in city treatment programs have been IV drug abusers in the past five to seven years and two thirds of them shared needles. ADAPT estimates that 80 percent of male IV drug abusers are dating females who are not drug users. These are just a few random indications of the extent of the ever-expanding reservoir of infection that is spilling over into the hospital.

Dino heard about ADAPT from his younger brother, who also has AIDS. People from ADAPT visited Dino's brother in jail on Rikers Island, where he's still being held in spite of his illness. Recently another of Dino's brothers, a drug dealer, was shot in his apartment, in his bed, in his sleep. The funeral was last week. "My *other* brother was killed the same way, man," Dino says. Dino shakes his head. "So my brother with AIDS came to the funeral. He was there. He was in handcuffs. He had to go right back."

This afternoon there are 26 inmates in the "AIDS cellblock" on Rikers. The connection between drugs and incarceration has long been taken for granted—last year four in ten indictments right here in the Bronx involved drug use—but the connection between prison and AIDS is new. Of the 50,000 inmates who passed through Rikers Island last year, as many as 12,000 were thought to be infected with the HIV virus. AIDS is now the leading cause of death among prisoners in New York State.

Dino and Mr. Flores have both been in prison, too, and when Mr. Carter leaves to photocopy the newsletter, they sit quietly swapping stories about what it was like. Mr. Flores, a nervous, powerfully built man, maintains that prison was a good experience. Partly because there's a reporter in the room, partly because he wants to believe it, Mr. Flores delivers a jeremiad on the benefits of incarceration. Speaking in a hard, flat voice, he tells how good prison was for him, how he spent five years in prison just thinking, how he pulled himself together in prison, and how he is going to pull himself together now.

Dino pretends to listen but his eyes are blank. He twiddles his thumbs. His hair and beard are streaked with gray. He is 41. He has been a drug addict for 30 years.

Mr. Flores is hopeful about his prognosis. He is "building up my antibiotics" through diet. He is taking the new drug called AZT. He has developed a rash from it, but aside from that—so far, so good. They said AZT might make him anemic but he feels good. Mr. Flores hopes AZT is a wonder drug that will save his life.

Dino is not on AZT. He had to stop taking it "on account it killed my blood cells." He has a lot of complaints to voice today. "I'm beat, man. I get exhausted. I get exhausted just walking the five flights up to my apartment. I get attitude, too. Sometimes I just shut myself up in the bedroom and sleep, you know? I don't go out. I'm jumpy. I get attitude from nothing. My son, he comes in from school and he throws down his books, I blow up. I never used to do that. It's this thing man"—he does not say AIDS.

(Last week, when Mr. Lares, eyes bulging in a sallow face, complained that the clinic gave *him* attitude because he never saw the same doctor twice, Dino told him he had "a hostility problem.")

It isn't good, Dino says. If the weather were warm, he'd be outside selling name bracelets. He sets up a table on the street in the spring and pretty soon word gets around that the name-bracelet man is back. Dino says it's the only time he's happy, when he has a pair of plyers and some wire in his hands. "I'm good at it. I make good money at it. I once had my own flea market. Everyone knows me. Howya-doin?"

Harold Campbell comes into the room, mutters a word of greeting, and gravitates toward the corner.

Mr. Flores has taken off his leather cap and is twirling it in his hands.

"I just hang around the house," Dino continues, speaking to no one in particular. "My wife, she's a diabetic. She's sleeping with the baby now."

"I'm doing good," insists Mr. Flores.

"I'm running up twelve flights of stairs every day in the projects where I live," says Mr. Campbell from his corner. Mr. Campbell has ARC—though no one here is exactly clear on why that makes him different. Mr. Campbell's legs and wrists are covered with a rash that makes his brown skin black as charred marshmallow. His hands look as if he's been working in a garage. Because his wife and two girlfriends have died of AIDS, Mr. Campbell says, the children in the projects call him "girl killer." Because of this rash, he says, people on the street fall back when he passes "like I'm a walking plague."

Mr. Carter returns with copies for everyone of the ADAPT newsletter. "These are good people," Dino says, tapping the sheets of paper in his hand. The cover of the newsletter bears a crude illustration of a big hypodermic needle and a pile of skulls. "Before these people got on the case, the brothers with this at Rikers was all in a room where everybody coughed all over everybody else. Now they change the sheets every day, not once a week, and they got screens between the beds."

"I'm going to the dermatology clinic tomorrow," Mr. Campbell says from his station in the corner.

"That's great, man," Dino replies absentmindedly. Dino can barely drag himself up the stairs to his apartment. This guy says he's taking them two at a time.

The door opens and Milagros Fuentes slips in with Richie Suarez on her heels. Neat, trim, her face carefully painted, Milagros is almost 40 but looks years younger. Milagros has AIDS but she looks great. She is also taking the new wonder drug, AZT. Richie, 32, is her lover. Richie has ARC and has been in the hospital once because of it. Now, he says, he feels fine—he makes it clear today, he's just along for the ride, to keep Milagros company.

Most of the time, Richie lives at Milagros's apartment. When they argue, which is frequently, Milagros accuses Richie of giving her AIDS, and Richie screams back that she gave it to him. Since Richie found out he had ARC, he's overdosed on pills twice—both times, he's downed them ostentatiously in front of Milagros.

Richie is tall, handsome, dark skinned, well dressed, well spoken. He has a black mustache. Black moles are scattered over his throat and face. You immediately think, he is the kind of man who as a boy lived in a house with a lot of sisters darting back and forth, waiting on him.

The men stumble over themselves to offer a chair to Milagros. Since Connie Rivera stopped coming to clinic—maybe she's better, maybe too sick—Milagros is the only woman in the group and she receives due deference. There is no discussion about sex and/or condoms in front of Milagros.

(When guilt over her supposed frigidity goads Milagros into approaching Richie again, in a few weeks, she will be surprised to learn that he won't have sex with her without using a condom—this, she will tell him, is proof that he doesn't really love her.)

Demure, dignified, self-contained, Milagros doesn't say much, so everyone was surprised last week when, with a little prodding, she told a long story about a fight she had with her daughter. She'd sat mute for an hour and when Mr. Carter asked her if she wanted to say anything, Milagros said, "No, but listening makes me feel sadder. I get a lump in my chest like I want to cry."

"Why do you want to cry?"

Then Milagros burst forth with her story:

Milagros has two daughters, 12 and 15. The older one has always been a problem. This daughter lives in Washington, D.C., with her boyfriend, who is no good. This daughter came to New York to see her mother and told Milagros she was pregnant.

"You're not pregnant," Milagros insisted. "I know you just had your period."

Her daughter screamed, "You don't believe me, I'll kill myself!"

Milagros's daughter said she was going to get a knife from the kitchen and stab herself. There was a struggle. Milagros wrestled her daughter to the floor. She pulled her down by the hair—somehow she found the strength. They wrestled on the floor. Slowly Milagros's daughter dragged herself and her mother across the floor into the kitchen. In the kitchen Milagros's daughter seized a butcher knife and held it to her belly.

"I'll kill myself!"

Milagros reached for the knife. It slashed her hand. There was a lot of blood. Then, talking in a quiet voice, Milagros managed to get her daughter to drop the knife.

The two women fell into each other's arms, hugging and weeping. Sitting on the floor, Milagros spoke to her daughter about God and the Bible. But when her daughter tried to kiss her, Milagros froze and turned her face away, afraid she would give her AIDS.

Later when Milagros found the 12-year-old trying to mop up the blood on the kitchen floor, she yelled at her and chased her out of the room. Then she cleaned up the blood herself.

Today when she's asked about her daughter, Milagros says she went back to Washington. Milagros doesn't like to see her daughter living with this boyfriend, who has been in trouble with the police and who her daughter says seduced her when she was 11. But today Milagros says, "I don't care. She can stay there. We're fighting so much."

Everyone feels for this poor lady who never shot drugs but now has AIDS.

Milagros has not told the group that when her husband left her alone with two children and she lost her job and faced eviction, she turned to prostitution. For only one year, Milagros says, early in the morning, five days a week, she transformed herself from a whore back into a housewife on the subway home to her sleeping children. Milagros is able to admit now that she probably was first exposed to the HIV virus by a john, not by Richie. She is convinced that AIDS is a punishment from God for the things she did.

Dr. Lieberman comes to fetch Milagros. When they've left the room, Richie tells everyone what a bitch Milagros has been lately.

"She's a ball-buster," he says quietly. "She gets bitchy then she gets down on herself like she's nothin. I don't know."

"You don't look so good, man," Dino says. "What's wrong which-you?"

Beads of perspiration dot Richie's forehead.

Richie is in a methadone program in Harlem but his dosage is a low one. Some days he goes in and just pretends to drink the drug—he throws it away with the cup. He's still shooting heroin.

"You carry your own spike?" Dino asks.

Richie nods.

"You carry your own works, too? Without you carry your own cooker, you may as well be passing the needle."

Dino is fatherly, protective. He speaks as if Richie weren't already infected.

"I'm going off meth' anyway," Richie says. "I'm going back to P.R."

"You better cut down gradual and then you tell them you wanna detox, they'll send you to downtown. They'll give you the number of the doctor. You'll check in for 21 days and they'll detox you. But then you have to be willing not to get high."

At that, Richie smiles—his first real smile—and rolls his eyes. You see the child he was once. You see he will never go to detox.

Everyone laughs.

"I know," Dino says. "I done it. All that pain and sacrifice, then you're back on the street and you think, Just a little methadone would take the edge off of this. And you're right back where you started. The methadone, it's worse than horse." Dino is relentless. "Once I got these abscesses, you know? I got one on my neck out to here. I thought I was growing another head!" He laughs, a short bark, and passes a hand over his eyes. "I got one here, on my forehead. When the doctor cut it open, man, he said I had a garbage disposer in there. It was full of worms and shit. That didn't stop me. I was still shootin then."

During Dino's story, a tiny brown man, emaciated, is brought to the door by the receptionist. It's cold out today but the little man is wearing nothing heavier than a short-sleeved polo shirt over a T-shirt. His fly is undone. He is complaining of a headache. Mr. Carter takes him aside and does an intake interview on the spot. His name is Francisco Santos. He has trouble remembering how to say his social security number in English.

4. IS THERE ANYONE WHO LOOKS THAT PEACEFUL?

Fran Whelan's office, the Catholic chaplain's office, is a little cubicle with dirty red wall-to-wall carpeting. It's on the second floor of the hospital, down the hall from the chapel. It's quiet up here. There are a few straight-backed chairs and two somewhat battered metal desks in the room. There is a framed poster of the Virgin on the wall. When Sr. Fran finds herself spending a lot of time in this office, doing paperwork, she knows she is in mourning. She's avoiding the wards upstairs. She used to feel embarrassed and guilty about this. Now she allows herself room to grieve.

Sr. Fran is a member of the Dominican Sisters of the Sick Poor, a religious congregation founded in New York in 1872. An Irishwoman named Mary Walsh, who did laundry, was going to work one day when she saw a little girl crying in a doorway. Following the child upstairs, Mary Walsh found a sick woman in bed with a dead baby beside her. Mary Walsh's life was transformed by this event. She quit her job and devoted herself to the poor. She gained followers. They banded together. They took in laundry. They used the money they made to help poor

171

families, setting aside a little bit for themselves. They vowed to live a very simple life.

A small woman in her fifties, Sr. Fran is a trained nurse and has a degree in social work. It has been part of her religious vocation to work in a variety of settings in and around New York City—as a public health nurse, in a mental health clinic, in a well-baby program—always with the poor. A few years ago, Sr. Fran's congregation of some three score sisters went through a self-evaluation. If you could start all over again, its members were asked, what would you do? Sr. Fran decided she should go for pastoral training. Women were not then allowed to be Catholic chaplains in hospitals but they were permitted to carry out analogous functions. Sr. Fran got a job in pastoral care at St. Clare's Hospital in midtown Manhattan. That's where she first saw AIDS.

She first heard about it early in 1981. There was no name for it. She saw patients at the hospital who began to conform to a certain profile—they were all young men, they were all gay, and they all suffered from a wasting syndrome. For the most part, their disease went unacknowledged by the medical staff, who would treat them summarily for "undiagnosed allergies" or "white blood count trouble" and quickly discharge them. It slowly emerged that these patients all were suffering a loss of immunity.

It was Sr. Fran's goal to work in a municipal hospital but it didn't seem possible for a long time. Then in 1982, she heard about an opening for an office aide here. She applied for the job. Later, when the church decided to permit females to be chaplains, she approached the hospital administration and said, "I'm doing chaplain's work and have church approval—I need a chaplain's salary."

When Sr. Fran trained as a social worker, she was taught not to get involved with clients beyond a certain point. Pastoral work, she says, is different. You must care.

You must make yourself available as a person. You get hurt. That's part of the price you pay.

Sr. Fran visits patients and talks to them. She tries to lend support to their families. She helps in ways that sometimes seem insignificant—turning a patient over or getting a glass of water.

Getting a glass of water. It sounds like so little.

And many of the people she works with are so manipulative and so demanding, she sometimes finds herself hearing only the manipulation and not the desperate plea behind it, of somebody half her age who is dying and is really terrified to ask for anything whatsoever.

Get me a glass of water.

Around the time that Sr. Fran first came to this hospital, one of the social workers was organizing a bereavement program aimed at women with stillbirths. Often these women left the hospital without any follow-up. Often the social worker found that one of the first questions they asked themselves was, Why did God do this? So Sr. Fran was asked to join the program.

In the beginning, they worked with mothers who had stillbirths—and sometimes with fathers, too—but after a while they found they were drawing too strict a line. There were women who had lost a baby but it was termed an abortion because of the fetus's weight, so they were excluded, which seemed unfair. There were newborns who had taken one or two breaths. There were babies who had lived in the hospital one or two weeks. The program was reorganized to encompass all of these and its name was changed to "Paranatal Bereavement."

There are almost 4,000 births a year in the hospital. When babies are born dead, the mother is given the baby's footprints, urged to name the child, and urged to talk about the death. There is also an emergency burial fund for infants—Sr. Fran obtained the grant for it.

If the babies aren't buried privately, they're buried on Harts Island in Long Island Sound. Usually the bodies are taken from the hospital morgue to Jacobi Hospital, also in the Bronx, where they're put in boxes. Each box has a number on it and the name of the mother. The boxes are loaded on a truck and the truck travels by barge to Harts Island.

Because she wanted to be able to describe it to the women whose babies were buried there, Sr. Fran went to Harts Island one day. The burial ground is an open field with granite stones regularly spaced across it, square stones with numbers cut into the tops of them. A road runs through the middle of the field. Adults are buried on one side of the road, babies on another.

The day Sr. Fran visited Harts Island, prisoners from Rikers were digging graves. When they found out why she was there, one said, "You just tell those women we give those babies all the respect that we know how." Another said, "Tell them there are flowers growing here." Another said, "Tell them you can hear the ocean from where they're buried."

Sara's baby died almost a year before she did. It was spring. After the baby was born, Sara was discharged from the hospital but the baby stayed behind in intensive care. Sara had been on drugs. She still was. She visited the baby and saw it in the incubator a few times. When the baby died they had trouble locating Sara.

The day Sara came to see her dead baby, the social worker asked Sr. Fran if she would help. In the mortuary there are a bassinet and clothing people have donated. Sara, Sr. Fran, and the social worker laid out the baby and dressed her.

It was a baby girl. Sara had not even held her.

They dressed the baby in a pale green dress with smocking and embroidery on the yoke. Sara gave the baby a name. They said a prayer for the baby. Then Sara asked if she could hold it. She held it—not over her shoulder, but up, to look at it. They all cried.

They took Sara's picture with her baby.

Sara was about five-foot-three. She was very thin. She had freckles and long straight brown hair. She had big brown eyes. She was very near-sighted and wore glasses. Some of her teeth were missing.

Sara enjoyed clothes. She loved vivid colors. She knew where to buy designer clothes at discount in very small sizes. She loved food. She enjoyed life.

She had a delightful personality. Everyone she met was entranced. Social workers and psychologists, even nurses from her methadone program, adored Sara and went out of their way to do things for her. They would find themselves doing things for Sara they would never do for another client.

People would do things for her?

Yes, myself included.

Sara was artful. She had a way of asking questions about you to keep you interested. She would remember what you liked and where you were yesterday. She had an intense way of looking at you—not just weighing what you were doing now but calculating how it fit into what you might do next. There would be this way of asking, then watching to see, Is it working?

After Sara died, Sr. Fran met her sister and the sister said that meeting Sara late in life was like meeting another person from the one she grew up with. They were like two different people. If Sara hadn't reminded her of some of the things they'd done together when they were children, her sister wouldn't have recognized her. Sara had changed her way of speaking, dyed her hair, cultivated a carefree manner at odds with their strict Catholic upbringing.

Sara ran away from home in her teens. She took heroin and cocaine. She was a prostitute. She did time on Rikers Island. She got a black eye there for refusing to have sex with a guard. She and her pimp, The Old Man, lived flamboyantly. They were very showy. They dressed in the same color.

She had a number of relationships with men. She gave up two babies for adoption. After she went on methadone, then, she had three children, two girls and a boy. For a while she lived with a man named Stanley and shared needles with him. Stanley beat her, so Sara left him and took the children to a shelter. Stanley was the father of the baby girl who died.

Sara saw Stanley again when he checked into the hospital with AIDS during one of her stays there. Stanley died in Montefiore Hospital in March 1986.

Sara loved her children. She was good with children. She had a good grasp of their development and their needs. By the time Sr. Fran met Sara, she had made a home for them.

There was Sara, not long out of the hospital, obviously very ill. They all thought the first thing was to get Sara back into the hospital but they had a terrible time doing it. They tried to get her in through the emergency room but she didn't have the patience for it. Someone crossed her and she walked out. She was, of course, terrified to find out that what she suspected was true—that she had AIDS. But on one visit she gave them permission to run a blood test on her. She was positive for the HIV virus.

Once they got her into the hospital but she had an argument with somebody on the floor and disappeared.

Sara was still shooting drugs. She had a strong habit. She was taking at least 80 milligrams a day of methadone alone. She was not about to check into the hospital until she knew she'd get her methadone there. And she knew from being on the street what AIDS meant. So she took her time doing the things she had to do before she came in.

She gave up her children to foster care.

Sara finally checked into the hospital to stay in June.

When Sr. Fran heard she was there, she went up to visit her. All the people who knew Sara flocked to her room.

Sara made friends to survive. Getting her methadone, for instance, was a big event in her day. If she didn't get it on time, she would get cramps and pains in her joints. The longer it got delayed in the morning, the sicker she got and the longer it took her to get over it. So Sara made friends with the nurses. When they came on the floor in the morning, Sara would meet them and ask them to give her her methadone early.

Sara was in the hospital to build up her weight but they did a lung biopsy and found she already had *pneumocystis* pneumonia, so they treated her for that. She was in the hospital but she was still shooting drugs. Around 5 p.m., there is a change of shift and the staff is busy giving medicines. Sara would put on a coat over her pajamas, sail out the door, walk up to Third Avenue, buy the stuff, and come back.

Now Sara was homeless. Cured of *pneumocystis*, she had to stay in the hospital until the Department of Social Services found her a room in a hotel downtown near Times Square. A taxi service took her back and forth to her methadone program every day.

Sara didn't like the hotel. The neighborhood was strange and sometimes she was so disoriented, she would lose track of what day it was. So when she started feeling better, she sought out The Old Man, who lived in the Bronx. He owned his own home. Sara moved in with him. She was feeling better. She'd pulled herself together. She came to the outpatient clinic at the hospital regularly.

During this time, Sr. Fran kept in touch with Sara. One day in August, she even took Sara out to lunch.

Sara appeared at the door of Sr. Fran's office high as a kite, but pleasantly so.

They walked to an Italian restaurant not far from the hospital. Sara was stylishly dressed—she always dressed up to the minute. Sr. Fran wears somber skirts and sweaters, plain patterned blouses, but Sara loved to give her advice on clothes. Sara never missed a chance to tell Sr. Fran whether she looked good or not and she gave Sr. Fran her opinion walking to the restaurant that day.

"That looks nice with that."

When they sat down at the table, strangely enough, Sara was talking about contagion—reassuring herself by telling Sr. Fran how foolish it was for people to be afraid of catching AIDS when there had to be an exchange of blood and so forth. Bread was set on the table and Sara took a piece out of the basket. For example, Sara continued, no matter how many patients with AIDS Sr. Fran saw in the hospital—well, she'd have to have an open cut to catch AIDS from one of them, wouldn't she? Even then, she probably wouldn't catch it. People were funny. Sara broke the bread in two and handed a piece to Sr. Fran. Sr. Fran took the bread, and she realized, she was afraid to eat it. Of all people. She was not as free of prejudice as she'd thought she was.

Sara came back into the hospital, with *pneumocystis* pneumonia again, in September. Sr. Fran visited her room often. She was attracted to Sara. She enjoyed being with her.

Sara told Sr. Fran about the hurts she'd received from the Catholic Church when she was a little girl in parochial school—how when her mother couldn't afford the tuition, she took her children with her to see the nun to ask if they could postpone the payments, and the nun said no, and her mother cried so. Sara said she never forgot that.

There are always a lot of people circulating through the hospital promoting different creeds, and one of them told Sara she must pray constantly.

"Now why would you want to do that, pray always?" she asked Sr. Fran.

"What do you think?"

"I don't think that's what God wants us to do. I think

you're supposed to enjoy life and, like, know God is there."

Walking down Broadway one day, on impulse, Sr. Fran bought Sara a nightgown. It was wild. It was purple.

Sara was in and out of the hospital. She always had lots of friends on the ward. She was especially close to one man—Raphael Hernandez. He'd been in the hospital with ARC a long time. Anyway, Raphael said, he couldn't return to Puerto Rico because he'd shot someone and they were looking for him. Sara and Raphael would sit in the dayroom and talk and smoke cigarettes. Raphael had been on drugs a long, long time, too. People teased Sara and Raphael and said they were a hot number.

The Old Man visited Sara religiously. He was an avuncular kind of person, quiet, in his early fifties.

Sara was out of the hospital before Thanksgiving, back in before Christmas.

Sara avoided talking about death. When a boy she knew on the ward died crying out in pain, it frightened her. But deep down, Sr. Fran thought, Sara felt she would pull through. She talked as if AIDS were much more fatal on the street, as if being in the hospital afforded her special protection. She told Sr. Fran that people on the street with AIDS were staying out of the hospital longer than they should because they knew what was going to happen in the end and they wanted their freedom.

Even so, Sr. Fran sensed a kind of letting go in Sara. One day Sara mentioned Mother Teresa. "Is there anyone on earth who looks that peaceful?"

"What would you do if you met her, Sara?"

"Oh, I don't think I ever would."

But Mother Teresa came to the hospital on Christmas Day.

Fran went up to fetch Sara.

"Time to go to church."

"I don't think I want to go."

"Oh yeah, you do."

"No, I don't think so."

"You really do want to go, Sara."

So Mother Teresa came and talked to all of the patients and Sara was right up front.

She left the hospital against medical advice the next day.

Around this time, Sara's little boy, Aaron, was tested for AIDS at King's County Hospital in Brooklyn and found positive for the HIV virus. He was three and a half. The two little girls, six and eight, were in a foster home. When Sara returned to the hospital after New Year's, she began to fret about her children. "I can't do any more for my kids," she would say. She had kept phone numbers in a notebook—her social worker, Aaron's social worker, the social worker for her two little girls, the agency. She talked about putting her children in God's hands.

Sara got weaker. Her muscles were deteriorating. She fell out of bed. She could barely walk. She tried to use a walker but was too weak. Finally she was confined to a wheelchair.

It was arranged for the girls to visit and they came, accompanied by a worker from the foster-care agency. Sara was brought down in her wheelchair to Sr. Fran's office, where they could say good-bye in private. Sr. Fran had set out coloring books and crayons. She suggested to the agency worker that they step outside.

"Is it all right? Can they touch her?"

"Why don't you come with me and we'll let Sara visit with the children here."

The children stayed half an hour.

After a certain point, Sara couldn't hold up her head. A CAT scan showed that the trapezius muscles across her shoulders had broken down. They gave her a brace to wear but she refused. She was too proud. At the end, when she was comatose, they had to prop Sara's head up on the pillows so the weight of it wouldn't cut off her airway.

One day Sr. Fran went up to see Sara. She just lay there like a one-hundred-year-old person. It seemed to have happened overnight. When Sr. Fran talked to her, Sara made some noises but her gaze was fixed. There was no recognition after that.

She slipped—to me it was like someone falling off a hill.

Sr. Fran sat with Sara and held her hand and told her how much she was going to miss her.

After that, Sr. Fran found it hard to go back.

Sara Rojas died in the hospital on February 8, 1986. She was 32. In death, as in life, she managed to bend others to her will. Sara had a church funeral with a full mass, and her sister, a dental hygienist, quit her job in order to care for Sara's girls, whom she later adopted. No one in the hospital can say what happened to Aaron.

Sr. Fran lives in East Harlem. She shares an apartment with a group of other religious women who also work with the poor. One woman works with women prisoners, another is an educator for school dropouts, another is a visiting nurse. The apartment is above a social club where men play cards and gamble all day.

Last night, as she often does, Sr. Fran walked home from the hospital. She isn't afraid. She doesn't take chances.

When it snows, the avenues are spread with salt. On winter nights like last night, when the wind blows, a residue of salt and dust swirls up off the street. The acrid dust and salt get into your eyes and nose.

Last night, nearing 125th Street, Sr. Fran smelled another smell, something peculiar, and soon she came upon the charred wreck of a van, the kind with a luggage rack that shuttles to the airport and back. The driver, she learned later, had burned to death in the van, but the body was no longer there. The wind was blowing the white powder from the fire extinguishers into her face and that's what she'd tasted.

A glass of water. It seems like so little.

Sometimes Sr. Fran comes home laden with grief, so it's good that she doesn't need to explain a lot to the women she lives with—that someone died who was on a respirator for six days, had *pneumocystis* pneumonia, or whatever. She just needs to be able to say it's been a tough day, that she lost someone.

One Sunday when she didn't feel like working, Sr. Fran visited a young man dying of AIDS. He was very weak. His mouth was caked with secretions and he couldn't talk, so she put on gloves and wound her hands in gauze and cleaned out his mouth, cleaned off his tongue and the side of his face. No one had bothered to do that. He thanked her.

He said, "You take time."

"Yes, I do want to take some time with you."

"I think I'm dying."

"Who would you like with you?"

"My mother."

Sr. Fran doesn't talk to patients about God in dogmatic terms. Her message is a simple one about providence and accompaniment. You are not alone. Sr. Fran tells Bible stories without the traditional characters—the story of the loving father who waited and watched. Simple messages. I will not leave you. You are not alone.

5. TWICE DEATH

February 19. Mr. Carter goes up to 8-B to visit Jorge Torres. When Mr. Torres came into the hospital he had a place to live and a job. Now he has neither. By the time he was ready to go home in November, he had lost his room in the rooming house where he was staying because he hadn't paid his rent. Miraculously, another room was found and he was sent home in January with a cane. He came back to the hospital a week later. He is too weak to live alone. Mr. Carter asks Mr. Torres if he would like to transfer to Bird S. Coler Hospital on Roosevelt Island. Mr. Torres says yes.

Carmen Marcos is admitted to 9-A today. It is not her first admission. A sweet woman with a large, ever-present family, Mrs. Marcos says she got AIDS from her husband, who died of it. She weighs 59 pounds now. Her legs are like chair legs.

Dr. Lieberman visits Roberto/Roberta Cintron on 9-B. He seems sentient, but he will not respond. The CAT scan X-ray machine is out of order, so Dr. Lieberman can't properly evaluate him for toxoplasmosis. She prescribes medicine for toxoplasmosis anyway.

* * *

February 20. Mr. Carter phones the admissions office at Bird S. Coler Hospital about a transfer for Mr. Torres. They request that Mr. Torres bring copies of his CAT scans with him. His chest X-rays can come later.

Mr. Carter holds his inpatient group—patients willing and able to attend are brought to the ninth-floor dayroom. At 24, Jesus Gomez is the youngest patient with full-blown AIDS in the hospital. When Mr. Carter suggested the group to him, he responded enthusiastically, saying he needed to talk about his illness. But in the group he was silent and when Mr. Carter asked him why, he said, "Well, I'm not sure I have AIDS."

Alberto Flores, one of Dr. Lieberman's outpatients, calls her from a pay phone to say he has a rash but his money runs out and he gets disconnected. She can't call him back as he has no phone of his own. His white count is up now and Dr. Lieberman would like to put him back on AZT.

(Two weeks ago, in group, Mr. Flores said, "The way people treat you, this AIDS is twice death.")

Mrs. Marcos's eyes are veering, so in the evening Dr. Lieberman places her first in line for the CAT scan, which is still out of order.

Eighteen days after being placed in the intensive care unit, Rosalie Thomas dies. She is 40 years old.

(Next week, at Ms. Thomas's funeral, two of her brothers will get into a fight and one will kill the other. A nephew will be found wandering naked on the Grand Concourse the next night. A member of the family will tell Dr. Gerais that Ms. Thomas's nephew has been acting strangely since last May, when his father died of AIDS, and it looks like the funeral pushed him over the edge.)

February 21. On 9-B, Dr. Gerais talks to Royal Washington, the man who keeps his money in his socks. When Mr. Washington came into the hospital, he was drunk and delirious. He has cryptococcal meningitis, tuberculosis, fever, chills, and wasting syndrome. "You know," he tells Dr. Gerais, "I want to talk to Dr. Robinson, you know? And then there's Dr. Robinson right in front of me and I can't talk to him because I've forgotten what I wanted to say."

On 9-A, Dr. Gerais visits Delia Rosario. Just a few days ago, Ms. Rosario was psychotic, so Dr. Gerais prescribed some medication. Now Ms. Rosario lies docilely in bed. Dr. Gerais tries to have a conversation with her, but all Ms. Rosario wants to talk about is cigarettes.

"Wanna cigarette."

"I'm sorry, I don't smoke. I don't have any cigarettes. How do you feel today?"

"Wanna cigarette."

Dr. Lieberman learns that a specimen sample of Ms. Rosario's spinal fluid was lost on its way to the lab. The family refuses to permit another spinal tap. It's the kind of thing, Dr. Lieberman tells a colleague, that you want to scream about, but if you started screaming, you'd never stop.

Dr. Gerais visits Mr. Cintron on 9-B and finds him sitting up in bed. He seems to be responding to the medication Dr. Lieberman prescribed for toxoplasmosis. "I hear you were depressed, Roberta."

"Yeah, that's what everyone's been telling me but I can't remember. And you know me, Doctor—I'm not that way." (In a few weeks, still short of his goal, still a man, Mr. Cintron will die in the hospital.)

The CAT scan is broken.

February 22. Every time Mr. Carter looks in on little Mrs. Marcos, she's asleep. The CAT scan is still out of order so there is no way to know, but Mrs. Marcos probably has a massive lesion on her brain. Now she might not be rouseable. (Mrs. Marcos will die in the hospital in March.)

A rumor circulates that the hospital is going to be searched for drugs. One patient quickly vanishes.

February 23. Mr. Carter spends a lot of time photocopying the last two months of Mr. Torres's chart so he can take it with him when he gets transferred to Coler Hospital tomorrow. He makes arrangements with the ambulette service to have them drop by Mr. Torres's bank on the way to the hospital, so he can withdraw his savings.

Freddie Pagan comes to the emergency room and is admitted into the intensive care unit. He is immediately put on a respirator. He is a recovering addict, young, anxious. When Dr. Lieberman comes to see him, he grabs her hand. (Mr. Pagan will be ready to leave the hospital in April, but his stepmother, mother, and grandmother will refuse to have him, so he will remain hospitalized, homeless, indefinitely.)

The CAT scan is still broken.

February 24. It is sunny, clear, and cold today. In column two beneath the fold on the front page of *The New York Times,* there is a story by Thomas Morgan on AIDS in the workplace informing readers that 9,000 New Yorkers have been diagnosed with AIDS since record keeping began and that the city health department now lists AIDS as the leading cause of death among young men 25 to 44 and women 25 to 29.

In "Science Times," Lawrence K. Altman reports that a forum is about to begin in Atlanta to discuss issues surrounding the HIV antibody test—proposals, for instance, to make testing mandatory in certain instances. More than 36,000 Americans have been officially diagnosed with AIDS, Dr. Altman writes, and there are projections that by 1991 more than 50,000 cases could be diagnosed—each year.

There are 580 patients staying in the hospital today— children and adults occupying 512 out of 539 available beds, plus 68 newborns. More than half the newborns in the hospital are so-called "boarder babies" waiting for placement by foster care agencies. There are 28 adult patients in similar circumstances, waiting for transfer to facilities like nursing homes. Half of them are over 50. The youngest is 16, the oldest 88.

In the next 24 hours, 2,386 prescriptions will be dispensed. The kitchen will serve 2,779 meals—1,606 to patients, 1,173 to staff and visitors in the cafeteria. As of this afternoon, the billing department will be owed $2,112,635.50 for 3,888 patient days' worth of hospital services. The cashier's office will take in $482,435.31. Whether a patient is in the intensive care unit or on the ward, the daily billing rate is $694. Medicaid reimburses the hospital $578.20 per day; Medicare, $508.90; Blue Cross, $549.84.*

When the AIDS team meets this morning, there are 32 patients on the list. (Seven of them will die by the beginning of April.)

Florence Bayer died yesterday. "I couldn't stand it," confesses Dr. Gerais, "so I didn't even look in yesterday to see if she was still around. Over the weekend, I was wiping her tears away as I talked to her."

Abdul Husseni, who screamed so when they gave him a spinal tap, left against medical advice last night. "I just hope he comes to clinic," Dr. Lieberman says. "His white count dropped with no explanation but he wouldn't let us do a bone marrow test." (Mr. Husseni will die in another hospital.)

The CAT scan is still broken.

*On any given day, there are nearly 1,000 AIDS patients in New York City hospitals, so given rates like the above, it costs at least $600,000 per day to treat them. On the average, an AIDS patient in New York City is kept in the hospital 21 days, so each hospital stay costs at least $13,000 per patient. Last year, $400 million was spent citywide on medical costs resulting from AIDS.

A total of $1.1 billion was spent on AIDS in the U.S. in 1986 and around $7 billion was lost in earnings and employee output. The federal government will soon estimate that by 1991, $10–15 billion will be spent each year on medical and social services for people with AIDS.

Herman Quintero, cured of *pneumocystis carinii* pneumonia for now, will be discharged later in the day.

Miguel Lares will be admitted to the hospital this afternoon. Mr. Lares, who Dino says has "a hostility problem" because he constantly complains in the outpatient group, was diagnosed with *pneumocystis* over a year ago and has been in and out of the hospital three times.

By the end of the day, Luis Bonilla will be admitted with toxoplasmosis. By Thursday he will be unresponsive. (Mr. Bonilla will die in the hospital next month.)

Anna Maldonado will be admitted today to see if she has ARC. Her husband Cesar has AIDS and was admitted last Wednesday. Nurse Baez strong-armed Mr. Maldonado into telling his wife he had AIDS—he was still having sex with her without taking precautions.

Dino's brother will be admitted today. A few days ago the court suddenly reversed his sentence and he was released from Rikers Island.

Six patients are waiting to see if they have AIDS. (All will be diagnosed with AIDS.) Six other patients have ARC. (One of these will die from a combination of ARC and tuberculosis.)

Nine AIDS patients have as their primary infection *pneumocystis* pneumonia; five cryptococcal meningitis; four toxoplasmosis. Two patients are known to have both cryptococcal meningitis and toxoplasmosis. Two patients are suffering from chronic renal failure. Only one patient on the list has Kaposi's sarcoma.

Fourteen patients on the list are homeless or about to become homeless.

One patient who makes a rare appearance on the list this morning is an HIV-infected infant who has been in the hospital awaiting placement in a foster home for some time now.

At 10 a.m., Mr. Torres, a small man in his late forties with traces of eczema on his face, is pacing the halls on

8-B, anxious about his transfer this morning to Coler Hospital.

Mr. Torres is strong. He has survived cryptococcal meningitis and lymphoma. At one point between hospitalizations, Mr. Torres attributed his survival to Jesus. He had found Jesus, he preached in the outpatient group, and Jesus was going to save him. He said that he had found Jesus so he didn't need any medicine—he was only taking it so as not to tempt God.

When he came back into the hospital, though, Mr. Torres was angry and depressed. He felt Jesus had betrayed him. He also felt betrayed by Mr. Carter. For some time, Mr. Torres had been working as a volunteer in the admitting office and he'd applied for a paying job when word got around that he had AIDS. Although he was given the job, Mr. Torres seemed to think that Mr. Carter tried to block his advancement by leaking his diagnosis.

During this last stay in the hospital, Mr. Torres's disposition has improved. He's still angry at Mr. Carter, but in general, he has become more mellow, talkative, and cooperative. He doesn't talk about Jesus very often. The staff in Admitting grew very fond of Mr. Torres. Ms. Santiago, the director, says it marked a great change in her staff when they accepted Mr. Torres.

Mr. Torres's most recent hospital stay has lasted 44 days and cost Medicaid $25,440.80. The hospital will absorb a $6,000 shortfall.

But now the hospital seems reluctant to let Mr. Torres go. The request for copies of his CAT scans evidently never reached his doctor.

At 10:45, after the team meeting, when Mr. Carter comes onto the floor, Mr. Torres rushes up to him.

"What about my transfer, Mr. Carter?"

"I'm just checking."

The floor nurse tells Mr. Carter that Mr. Torres's papers have to be signed by the day administrator, who is holding up the release because Mr. Torres's CAT scans aren't among them.

10:50: To save time, Mr. Carter takes the stairs down to the seventh floor. He enters the day administrator's office.

11:10: Mr. Carter emerges from the day administrator's office.

11:15: On the phone in his own office, Mr. Carter is speaking to Coler Hospital. He explains that the request for the CAT scans never made it through the bureaucracy. The admitting nurse at Coler asks how long it will take to get the scans.

"At this point, I'm so frustrated and angry with the system that I don't know," Mr. Carter says.

The admitting nurse at Coler volunteers to take Mr. Torres without the CAT scans.

11:20: Mr. Carter rushes up the stairs to 8-B. The unit social worker shuffles through the release papers and says Mr. Torres can go as soon as they are photocopied.

"Did the ambulette come?" Mr. Carter asks.

"No, but Mr. Torres left," a nurse says.

"Left?"

"Yeah, maybe he went to church."

Mr. Carter leaves to search for Mr. Torres.

11:30: The ambulette driver appears, consults a piece of paper, and pushes a wheelchair down the hall to Mr. Tores's room.

It is a corner room, a single. The only sound in the room is the hiss of air through the baseboard air conditioner and the soft whirr of a floor polisher from outside in the hall. The sheets on Mr. Torres's bed are rumpled and stained. There is a brown smudge on his pillowcase. The call button, attached to its rubber cord, rests on the bed like a long white garter snake. The wastebasket is full of trash. Mr. Torres's lightweight jacket is draped over the arm of a chair. A white plastic shopping bag holding Mr. Torres's few earthly possessions sits on the windowsill.

"So where'd he go?"

11:40: Mr. Torres appears. He's been downstairs saying good-bye to his friends in Admitting. The social worker has returned with his papers and gives them to the driver. Followed by the ambulette driver, Mr. Torres walks to his room. Chatting with the driver in Spanish, he puts on his jacket and a beret. He picks up the shopping bag and sits down in the wheelchair.

Holding his bag on his lap, Mr. Torres is wheeled down the corridor. As he passes, a housekeeper in a blue uniform waves good-bye. At the nurses' station, the head nurse says, "Good-bye, Mr. Torres, don't abuse the privileges at Coler. They'll let you out on a pass but you have to come back on time."

Mr. Torres is wheeled down the hall and disappears around the corner.

At 11:50, Mr. Carter returns to the nurses' station and is told Mr. Torres has gone.

Mr. Carter feels a sinking sensation. He has known Mr. Torres—how long now? A year and a half? And he wanted to say good-bye.

6. ON HOLD

Noon. On 9-A, in room 61, Delia Rosario lies on her side in bed. Behind her, a black-and-white TV is playing. A flowering plant with wilting, blackened petals sits on a table against the wall. A plastic stake in the vase reads "Please Water Me, I'm Thirsty."

Ms. Rosario is a light-skinned black woman with short, tan hair. A sheet lies across her shoulders but one slender hand with long fingers extends from beneath the bedclothes. The fingers twitch now and again.

She has stopped asking for cigarettes. (Ms. Rosario will die eight days from now.)

Noon. On 9-A, in room 77, Mr. Santiago is still waiting for a visit from his wife.

Noon. On 4-D, in room 219, Albert Schult sits in a chair feeding Frederico Delgado out of a bottle and talking to him. The HIV virus was transmitted to Frederico in the womb by his mother. He has lived in the hospital since last June. He is two and a half years old.

Frederico's father, Hector, died from AIDS last September. His mother, Peggy, died from AIDS two months later. Now Frederico is a so-called boarder baby. He is "on hold," waiting for placement. He is one of about 300 children living in hospitals in New York City this afternoon because accredited foster homes can't be found for them. Frederico happens to be disabled—he was born with cerebral palsy in addition to his HIV infection—but children all over the city who have no handicaps or illnesses are in the same position.

Mr. Schult, Frederico's only visitor from the outside, comes to the hospital each week on Tuesdays and Sundays. Frederico's mother, a niece by marriage, was to Mr. Schult "the daughter I never had." When Peggy died, Mr. Schult was essentially her closest living relative. Her mother had died when Peggy was in her teens. A telegram was sent to her father's address in Florida—it was not returned but it wasn't answered either.

Frederico's father's mother has visited him once. His great-grandmother visited at Christmas. After Peggy died, Hector's family sent Frederico's five-year-old brother, Hector, Jr., to Puerto Rico to live with relatives there. But no one in Hector's family is willing to take Frederico.

Because he's spent over a year and a half in the hospital, Frederico has had more than his share of childhood illnesses. One of the nurses on his unit says Frederico "picks up everything—everything."

Dr. Aditya Kahl, Frederico's doctor, says his prognosis is "fair." It's hard to know. A large number of HIV-positive children—if they haven't also been infected with toxoplasmosis or cytomegalovirus in the womb—do well, particularly those who don't develop opportunistic infections within the first year. Children might actually have a special ability to overcome HIV infection. Frederico has had no opportunistic infections. His diagnosis is ARC.

Frederico can't sit up or stand. He can't hold a bottle. It's extra work to feed him and keep him clean. His eyes are severely crossed. When he was brought to the hospital, already bearing the label "HIV-infected," the doctors determined that Frederico was brain damaged. It's hard to know how much. It's possible he'll learn to talk, but since he has so little adult companionship, he hasn't had much of a chance to learn. Children need adults for growth and company. Generally, the hospital personnel do as well as they can but they're busy.

This week there are 471 children under 13 who have been officially diagnosed with AIDS in the U.S. As many as 2,000 have other illnesses related to HIV infection. The New York City health department estimates that 800 babies will be born in the city this year infected with the virus assumed to cause AIDS.

Since the fall of 1983, there have been one or two HIV-positive children in the hospital at all times. Their ages have ranged from infancy to five years old, although other hospitals have seen children as old as nine who were infected *in utero* with the virus. Dr. Kahl, a kindly man with an intense gaze, says that during the course of the epidemic he has "seen the best of it and the worst of it."

"What followed the arrival of the first child in the fall of 1983 was our growing-up period—a year or two of paranoia and fears. There was little information about transmission. Initially, the children were kept in isolation. People would glove and gown. There was much apprehension on all levels. But, happily, interactions changed. There is no isolation now, though we do realize that these children are at risk of infection themselves."

Standard infection control measures are observed in the pediatric section as they are all over the hospital.

"You have to live your own life," Dr. Kahl says philosophically, "and learn your own way. We've learned to live with the problem every day and we deal with it in a much more humane way now than we did the first year or so. It was sad the way the children were treated—not just here but in every hospital around the country—isolated and with a lack of compassion because of people's fears.

Some of it is still not the same as it would be for another
child, but that's changing for the better. What's happening outside—squabbles over children attending school,
day care, and so forth—is very upsetting. There are only
a handful of these children alive, not even that many of
school-going age. Now we know that casual contact bears
no risk, but the anger is still focused on the children.
That for me has been the worst part of the epidemic."

Sometimes the parents of other children on the unit
find out about children like Frederico and cause trouble.
"In this day and age," says Dr. Kahl, "everyone has an
opinion—doctors, nurses, transporters, IV-team people.
We have 60,000 types of workers in the hospital and they
all have opinions and they are at extremes all the time. So
parents do find out, off and on, and then there is a
certain amount of commotion. This is another reason for
keeping these children a little bit more protected."

Dr. Kahl has a special perspective on the tragedy of
AIDS. "For us—as opposed to a hospital in the city dealing with hemophiliacs and so on, one that is dealing with
intact families—there has been very little support. There
are no families in most of these cases. Even the federal
government has neglected the children until now. Everything has been directed almost totally toward adults. Almost nothing comes to kids. The children have borne the
brunt of the public's outcry and wrath."

Dr. Kahl says there has been nothing like this in the
developing world for 20 years—where a child is awake
and aware and dying like this. It is comparable to death
from polio or diphtheria. He sees two kinds of deaths
among children. The first involves the child under one
year who dies quickly, perhaps from *pneumocystis* pneumonia. That is like any other acute death. The second is
the child who "just slowly and literally withers away in
front of you over a period of weeks to months. That's the
very painful part. They're sick and dying over a long

period of time and you're not able to do anything about it."

Mr. Schult says he would come visit Frederico more often, but he's a night watchman for the parks department, so he comes home at 8 a.m. most days and goes to sleep. Mr. Schult is overweight. He has to rip the tops of his socks to accommodate red, swollen calves. He has Von Rickenhauser's disease—which is what the Elephant Man had. He is alone and growing old. His relatives are dying off. He wouldn't be able to take care of Frederico.

Frederico's mother Peggy was born in 1952, when Mr. Schult was a prisoner of war in Korea. Mr. Schult says he always had good rapport with Peggy. She had a wild temper and he was the only one who could handle her. "Her mother and father used to smack her across the face but I used to say to her, 'Now listen here, young lady, calm yourself down or I'll take you over my knee and paddle you.' "

Peggy, he says, was very beautiful. He has a photo of her in his wallet. The photo is of a smiling, attractive woman with a quintessentially Irish face. She is wearing slacks and a jersey printed with black and white stripes. Her hair is brown. "She had red hair but Hector made her dye it," Mr. Schult says, "because all the men were after her all the time."

Peggy was 34 when she died. She'd been an addict most of her life. "When she was sober, when she was straight," says Mr. Schult, "she was such a vivacious, fun-loving and giving girl. She was the kind of woman who would make any man a good wife, a good homemaker. But she got involved with the dregs of society."

Peggy was born in Connecticut. Later her family moved to Tampa. Mr. Schult says Peggy's parents were both alcoholic and beat her and her younger brother. Peggy once told him that her father had sex with her as well.

Peggy dropped out of high school and began to take

drugs. She was also involved in prostitution, in Florida and in Puerto Rico. Mr. Schult says that Peggy was attracted to light-skinned black men and Puerto Rican men but mainly attracted to men who could get her drugs.

When Peggy was 22, she came to New York City where she lived with Mr. Schult and worked at odd jobs. She took heroin and drank too much. Mr. Schult learned later that she also turned tricks when she lived with him.

In 1975, Peggy joined a methadone program and met a man named Charles Nadal. They both went straight. They moved to Atlantic City, New Jersey, together, where she worked in a hotel as a waitress. After two years in Atlantic City, Peggy had a fight with Charles and left him. She took the bus back to New York City and moved in with Mr. Schult again.

Peggy waited on tables at a restaurant near Columbia University. Mr. Schult says she was very popular there. "A cop was in love with her." She took in $60 to $70 in tips every day. She was doing well. But then, Mr. Schult noticed, she began staying out late at night, drinking, missing days at work. "I'm warning you," he told her, "that monkey's right over there in the corner waiting for you. You're going to goof up." She didn't listen.

Charles Nadal came back to New York. Peggy lived with him in a single-room-occupancy hotel for a while. In 1981, when they were still together, she entered a detoxification program run by Beth Israel Hospital. She met Hector Delgado in the program. They fell in love.

At one time, Mr. Schult says, Hector had been a restaurant cook. His family was upright. They were Jehovah's Witnesses.

Peggy and Hector never married. They were both on methadone. They were both on welfare. They lived in a city-owned apartment on Hough Avenue, near his family. Mr. Schult says Peggy kept house meticulously. She spent most of her days watching crime programs and situation comedy reruns on TV.

In 1982, Peggy gave birth to Hector, Jr. Frederico was born in October 1984. He was named after Hector's brother. The brothers were very close. Uncle Frederico was also a drug abuser and he died of AIDS soon after Frederico's birth—Mr. Schult doesn't know exactly when.

Frederico was born prematurely at Jacobi Hospital. Peggy had been drinking throughout her pregnancy and was on methadone as well. Frederico was treated for methadone withdrawal. He was also enrolled in Jacobi's neonatal "life program."

He was not a special problem. He ate some solid food and loved formula mixed with baby cereal. Perhaps he was a little cranky. Frederico has a mean temper, says Mr. Schult, like his mother.

In the spring of 1986, it became clear that both of Frederico's parents were dying from AIDS. They were both still drinking. Both had been on methadone for five years.

Peggy permitted doctors at Jacobi Hospital to test Frederico's blood. It was positive for the HIV virus. When she decided to go into a detoxification program in Yonkers, Peggy signed Frederico over to the Bureau of Child Welfare. A Bureau worker brought Frederico to the hospital on June 3, 1986. There was some discussion about an operation to fix his crossed eyes.

Peggy came to see Frederico in the hospital twice. Mr. Schult came to see him each week. When Mr. Schult tried to get Peggy to see Frederico more often, she would say, "Oh, he doesn't remember me."

Hector was dead on arrival at Jacobi Hospital on September 2, 1986.

(For years the toilet in Hector's and Peggy's apartment was broken and they had to pour water into it to make it flush. A week after Hector died, the plumber came to fix it.)

After Hector died, Peggy spent her days sitting in a chair in front of the TV, drinking. Right after he died, she had a couple move in with her. They were people she'd met hanging out, drinking, in front of a liquor store on Southern Boulevard. Peggy's friends supplied her with liquor and pills. Mr. Schult brought Peggy liquor, too.

Peggy was in mourning for Hector—"Hector, Hector, Hector."

"Hector was cheating on you," Mr. Schult reminded her, "fucking around with all these whores, hanging around with all the dregs of humanity, and you still love him?"

She would wail—"Don't talk about him that way!"

"You have to pull yourself together, think of your children."

Peggy was sinking fast so Mr. Schult took charge of Hector, Jr. Since Mr. Schult had no one to help him watch over Junior, he took him to work at night. Junior slept on a couch. At 7 a.m., he would wake up crying after three or four hours' sleep. Mr. Schult would take Junior home and put him to bed, then walk the dog, Spunky. Junior liked Spunky. He liked to pull Spunky's hair. But Spunky is old and would run under the bed.

Junior loved to ring the bell on the bus. "If you don't stop that," Mr. Schult warned him. "I'm going to take down your pants and paddle your bare bottom in front of all these people."

"Oh, don't do that."

But Junior was just like his mother. He couldn't resist ringing the bell. So Mr. Schult did what he'd threatened.

"Oh, look at his bare bottom," the people on the bus said.

By the end of October, it was evident that Peggy was going to die unless she went into the hospital. Her face had caved in. She was jaundiced. Normally fastidious, she'd been wearing the same shirt for weeks.

One evening, Mr. Schult says, he went to her apartment and told her, "The free ride is over, Peggy. I'm not buying you no more liquor. No more vodka, not even a drop. Forget about it. Let me dial 911 and we'll get you into the hospital then straighten things out when you get better."

She stared at him reproachfully. He'd always given her everything she asked for before. "Will they give me my methadone and something to help me detox right away?"

"Yes, they will."

He called the ambulance. By the time they got Peggy downstairs, they had to put an intravenous line in her.

In the hospital Peggy was sober. She seemed resigned to death. She wanted to say good-bye to her children. With the cooperation of a social worker from Peggy's drug program, Mr. Schult managed to get Junior in to visit. Mr. Schult talked to Peggy about God and said the Sinner's Prayer with her.

Peggy had been in Jacobi Hospital only three weeks when she died of cirrhosis, narcolepsy, and complications from AIDS. She was cremated and interred next to Hector.

A week after Peggy's death, Mr. Schult says, Hector's family called him.

"We want Junior."

"How about Frederico?"

"He's in the hospital. We want Junior now."

Mr. Schult says Hector's family doesn't think Frederico is Hector's son "because he's so light." But he has Hector's eyes.

This is the way Mr. Schult explains it—"They went through AIDS with his uncle, big Frederico, they went through AIDS with Hector, they went through AIDs with other members of the family." No one wants to go through AIDS with Frederico.

Hector's family took Junior to live with them. Later, Mr. Schult says, they asked him not to visit Junior so often because "he loves you too much." Every time Mr. Schult visited, they explained, Junior cried when he left.

Then, Mr. Schult says, Junior "was spirited off to Puerto Rico" by his grandmother and his aunt. "Maybe they thought he'd forget me if they sent him to Puerto Rico. But I don't think he will. I think he'll remember me."

Mr. Schult visits Frederico twice a week almost without fail. He feeds Frederico. Frederico won't eat solid food. When you try to get him to, he screams and spits it out. He has a mean temper. He likes his bottle, though. After Mr. Schult gives Frederico his bottle, he seats him in an infant carrier in his crib—it's better for Frederico's digestion. Soon Frederico will fall asleep.

When Mr. Schult first came to visit Frederico, the staff was suspicious—what's this old man doing, coming to see this baby?

Frederico is an exceptionally beautiful child. He is very fair, with translucent skin. You can see the violet veins through the skin of his eyelids. He has curly light brown hair.

There's a scab on Frederico's knee. He has a fungal rash on his foot—Frederico's always liable to have a rash somewhere, usually on the back of his head or his neck.

When Frederico sleeps, he breathes heavily. He expels little sighs. His eyelids twitch. His sleep is sometimes so deep, he doesn't wake up when he's spoken to or touched.

Sometimes Frederico has to wear mitts made of stretch-knit bandage material knotted at one end and fastened around his wrists with adhesive tape. This is to keep him from pulling out tubes—sometimes he has to be fed formula through a nasal-gastric tube taped to his cheek and nose, sometimes he has to be given antibiotics intravenously. The mitts are also to prevent Frederico from scratching himself. Frederico's fingernails are very long. The staff doesn't cut them. It's quite a job to cut a baby's nails as you're afraid of cutting the baby. Lots of mothers just trim the nails by biting them. Frederico plays with the knots inside his mitts.

Frederico can't sit up or stand. He can't hold a bottle. He has little motor control. He sometimes has spasms. He squirms around and can get his head stuck between the bars of his crib. He likes his hands. He spends lots of time looking at them—the doctors say his vision has compensated for his crossed eyes.

They've decided not to operate on Frederico—there are risks due to his HIV infection, the surgeons say, and an operation on a child with cerebral palsy isn't always successful.

Frederico seems fascinated by a loose thread hanging off the corner of the padding that runs around the edge of his crib. He will reach up and touch it.

Sr. Barletta, Frederico's patient advocate, has crusaded on his behalf. She has argued with authorities and submitted reams of paperwork to get him into a rehabilitation day-care program outside the hospital. Some people wouldn't be bothered—let him be. But Sr. Barletta believes Frederico deserves the fullness of life. Unfortunately, just when he was about to go to day care, Frederico got a temperature, so day care got postponed.

Room 219 is out of the way. It's an isolation room down the hall from the nurses' station. Not many people pass by its safety-glass windows, so Frederico doesn't see or hear much activity. Until recently, he was in a room even more remote, with another infant who had AIDS and died. Some of the hospital volunteers feed Frederico and talk to him but they can't be there all the time. The nurses do their best.

But then, other nurses are prejudiced—quietly so, but they act on their prejudice. When one of them was asked by Sr. Barletta why Frederico wasn't in a room where he'd get more stimulation, she said the other children's parents didn't want that. The question then was, How did the nurses know they didn't?

Stuffed animals are lined up at the head of Frederico's crib. A musical mobile of circus animals in primary colors is fastened to the headboard. A heart-shaped balloon with the words "I Love You" is tied to the rail. When he's in his infant carrier, Frederico faces a blank wall with a bed lamp on it and a red sign that says NO SMOKING/NO FUMAR. Lying on his back, Frederico sees a white acoustic-tile ceiling.

There are two things in the room from Frederico's former life. One is a large brown plush teddy bear. The other is a music box made out of cardboard and plastic in the shape of a portable clock radio, with a yellow plastic handle and a spring for an aerial. The music box is covered with scratches, pencil marks, and ballpoint pen marks. Most of the printed decoration has worn off the box. There are cartoon mice on the clock face. The clock hands turn when the music box is playing. The music box plays "Hickory Dickory Dock." Frederico recognizes the sound and turns his head toward it when the music box is playing.

EPILOGUE

———— ⚜ ————

Early in 1985, when I suggested an article to the editors of *The New York Times Magazine* on "the human cost of AIDS," most reporting on the epidemic was scientific in nature and people with AIDS were often portrayed as faceless victims. I wanted to show the devastating impact AIDS was having on individual lives. It had certainly had an impact on mine. I was pretty sure I was carrying the virus and I was terrified.

Plainly, some of my reasons for wanting to write about AIDS were altruistic, others selfish. AIDS was decimating the community around me; there was a need to bear witness. AIDS had turned me and others like me into walking time-bombs; there was a need to strike back, not just sit and wait to die. What I didn't fully appreciate then, however, was the extent to which I was trying to bargain with AIDS: if I wrote about it, maybe I wouldn't get it.

My article on Jim Sharp and Edward Dunn ran in the *Times Magazine* in May 1985. But AIDS didn't keep its part of the bargain. Less than a year later, after discovering a small strawberry-colored spot on my calf, I was diagnosed with Kaposi's sarcoma.

Ironically, I'd just agreed to write this book. The prospect suddenly seemed absurd and out of the question, but "Write it," my doctor urged without hesitation. And on reflection, I had to agree. I don't believe in anything like fate. And yet clearly, along with what looked like a losing hand, I'd just been dealt the assignment of a lifetime.

Needless to say, reporting on the epidemic from my particular point of view has had its advantages and handicaps, but they're perhaps not the obvious ones. If I felt a special affinity for Manuella Rocha, it wasn't in small part due to the fact that I recognized in her eyes the same thing I saw in my own mother's eyes the day I gave her the news about myself. If I was scared sitting for hours in an airless room with a bunch of addicts with AIDS, it wasn't because I was scared of *them*. It was because their confusion and rage were precisely what I was feeling myself. The journalist's vaunted shield of objectivity was of little use at times like those. On the contrary, what counted most in the long run—on this story at least—was not my ability to function as a disinterested observer, but my ability to identify with my so-called subjects.

Nevertheless, long after I began writing, I worried about the morality, and even the feasibility, of producing a documentary-style piece of reportage like the one I'd contracted for—that is, without literally putting myself into it, in the first person, so to speak. It wasn't until I returned to the transcripts of my original interviews with Jim Sharp that I realized Jim was now speaking for me, too. Jim's grief, his despair, his terror—they were mine, too. But Jim's special gift was for anger. Life-affirming anger was the lesson Jim taught me, and anger has enabled me to write about the ocean of pain that engulfs us without drowning in it.

When I met Jim, I have to confess, I could only see a dying man. A chasm separated me from him and all the other men with AIDS I interviewed. Even though they were gay, as I am, even though most of them were my

own age, even though after I left those interviews I had
to stop on the street to cry, each one of them remained
safely "on the other side of the fence" for me. But now,
for good or ill, there is no "other side of the fence" and
no safety.

When I first met Jim, I could only see a dying man.
Last summer in Houston, when Jim came to his front
door to greet me, I met myself.

A few months after my article on him ran in the *Times*,
Jim announced without fanfare that he was moving back
to Houston, accepting an old friend's longstanding offer
of a room and sanctuary. Since I'd first interviewed them,
there had been plenty of indications that Jim and Dennis
weren't going to be able to make a go of it, so I wasn't
surprised. Jim needed, he said, to be with people who
loved and understood him best.

On the morning of his departure, Jim called and asked
if I'd do him a favor. He had some parcels he needed to
ship to Houston. Could I take care of them for him? A
car service was going to drive him to the airport that
afternoon and he'd drop the boxes by my place on his
way out of town.

I met Jim at his apartment to say good-bye. The little
studio had taken on a distinctly Gothic flavor since I first
saw it. Dennis had brought some of his furniture out of
storage—dark, carved Germanic pieces that included
straight-backed chairs suitable for a rectory. A pewlike
bench with carved finials stood at the foot of the bed.
The funereal atmosphere was augmented by black walls.

The place was tidy. Jim was packed and ready to go.
We sat and talked a while, waiting for the car, both
avoiding saying what was really on our minds. I felt sad
for Jim.

"You know if you ever need anything whatsoever, I'm
as close as the phone."

"Sure, sure."

He didn't seem to believe it.

Jim watched through the shutters. At the appointed hour, the car pulled up across the street. The driver came in and picked up some bags. Jim insisted on carrying one himself.

We got everything into the car and, while the driver and I waited, Jim locked up. Crossing the street, he looked defeated and frail. He got into the back of the car. His cane, the one Dennis had given him for Valentine's Day, was at his side. I sat up front with the driver and gave him directions to my apartment.

We drove down Carmine Street, past the corner grocery where Jim bought his cigarettes—by the pack, as if that made them somehow less lethal—past the coffeehouse where Jim and I had once spent a pleasant hour without mentioning AIDS once, past Our Lady of Pompeii, past the pasta shop, the luncheonette, the bagel store. This was my neighborhood, too.

As the car turned up Sixth Avenue, I felt a need to memorize the scene before my eyes—pedestrians crossing the intersection against the light, the sun falling on the brick facades of the apartment houses, the olive-drab leaves on the trees. I turned in my seat to look back at Jim. He was staring out the window, in his own trance. I was sure I'd never see him alive again.

Soon after the *Times* article on him and Jim was published, Edward Dunn brought me a gift. It was a little teddy bear—a nice ginger-colored teddy bear with a gingham ribbon tied around its neck. Since I didn't collect toys, I didn't know quite what to make of it. But Edward explained to me that he often gave teddy bears to friends because they represented warmth and gentleness to him. Later, he asked me what I was going to name mine.

"I hadn't thought of naming it."

"Oh, you have to name him," Edward said.

"I don't know, what do you think?"

"I thought you might call him Robert."

Since Robert was the pseudonym we'd chosen for his late lover, I saw Edward's gift in a new light. I realized that after the grueling interviews I'd put him through, Edward was paying me an enormous compliment. He was, in a way, placing a share of Robert's memory in my hands."

That fall, after over 20 years in New York, Edward moved to Los Angeles, saying it was time to begin a new life. Perhaps grandiosely, I wondered if our interviews didn't play a part in Edward's decision to leave the city— that they'd served as something of a catharsis or a watershed.

Over the next year and a half, "Robert" sat on the bookshelf in the hall and only came down when the cat knocked him down. Every once in a while I'd find "Robert" on the floor, dust him off and put him back on the shelf. I felt vaguely guilty about "Robert." I was no longer in touch with Edward.

One gloomy Saturday afternoon, a month after I began visiting Lincoln Hospital, I interviewed Sr. Fran Whelan at her home in East Harlem. That day she told me about the child I've called Frederico and I asked if I could meet him.

"If you go up with me. Then the nurses on the floor won't get upset."

"Why would they get upset?"

"They would wonder who you are. And then, too, I had a seminary student working with me and she wanted to do something in pediatrics. She told me that when she didn't wear gloves and that kind of thing, when she'd just play with him, they'd get upset."

That next week, I went up to the fourth floor with Sr. Fran. Frederico was asleep. The room was dim.

I peered into Frederico's crib. He was wearing mitts that day because he hadn't been eating well and they'd had to insert a feeding tube into one nostril.

There was a din from the hall—children crying, conversation, slamming doors.

"Kids develop a high tolerance for noise," Sr. Fran commented. "If you're tired, you sleep."

I peered into the crib. I heard a ringing in my ears. I almost bolted out of the room. Somehow, I kept my two feet planted where they were on the floor.

I'd seen eyes unblinking from lesions. I'd spoken to deaf ears. I'd held the hand of the dying man. But nothing had prepared me for this.

I wanted to snatch Frederico out of his crib, snatch him up and run away, run away with him. It was horribly, cruelly clear that I wanted for him what I wanted for myself, and I was powerless.

Later, as I walked down the hall beside Sr. Fran, I struggled to retain my composure. I hadn't, of course, told anyone at the hospital that I had AIDS.

"It's good the nurse saw you with us," Sr. Fran was saying. "Now you can come visit him lots, whenever you like, and there'll be no questions." In her quiet way, Sr. Fran is a real snakecharmer. She knew I'd go back.

And I did, more than once. I held Frederico in my arms. He smelled like piss and baby powder and he was quite a handful. He squirmed in my arms. I was a stranger. He didn't know me. He wanted to be put down.

The day I first saw Frederico, when Sr. Fran was distracted for a moment, I took "Robert" out of the plastic bag I was carrying and set him down among the other stuffed animals in the crib. I knew Edward would approve. What I didn't know was that Edward had AIDS and would die before the year was out.

It's taken me months to write this. I'm afraid to finish this book. I'm afraid of what will happen next.

When I met Jim, all I could see was a dying man. The day he left New York, I was sure I'd never see him alive again. But I did see him again, in Houston last June. He lives in a modest bungalow house on a tree-lined street. He's something of a celebrity. Until recently, he served on the board of the local AIDS foundation and he spends lots of time every day on the phone, dispensing comfort and advice to other people with AIDS. Among his other distinctions, Jim is probably the only man with AIDS in Texas who's lived long enough to collect Medicare there.

A week after I got back from Texas, Mr. Schult called to tell me Frederico was dead.

Things had finally been looking up for Frederico. Sr. Barletta had finally gotten him into day care. The agency had finally placed him in a foster home. But on his second night outside the hospital, inexplicably, Frederico turned blue. By the time the ambulance arrived, he was dead. For some reason, the emergency medical service didn't even try to revive him.

I went to the funeral home. Frederico lay in a little coffin lined with swagged white satin. He was dressed in a blue playsuit with speedboats on it.

"You dressed him in a playsuit," I said to Mr. Schult.

"And now he's at play," Mr. Schult sobbed, at my side. "He's romping in heaven now with Jesus like he never was able to down here."

I held Mr. Schult's arm tightly until the sobbing passed. The coffin was too small for the top of catafalaque. You could see gouges and scrapes and scars in the wood in the parts the coffin didn't cover. I looked down at the body in the coffin, beyond help. I agreed aloud with Mr. Schult that Frederico was in heaven now because it seemed to make him feel a little better.

I don't know why, but I always thought Frederico would live.

New York City
December 1987